Resuscitation of the Newborn

Senior commissioning editor: Mary Seager
Editorial assistant: Caroline Savage
Production controller: Anthony Read
Desk editor: Claire Hutchins
Cover designer: Fred Rose

Resuscitation of the Newborn: A Practical Approach

David Drew MB ChB MRCP DTMH MRCPCH
Consultant Paediatrician, Manor Hospital, Walsall, UK
Honorary Senior Lecturer in Paediatrics, University of Birmingham, UK

Philip Jevon RGN BSc(Hons) PGCE
Resuscitation Training Officer, Manor Hospital, Walsall, UK
Regional Representative, Resuscitation Council (UK)

Margaret Raby RGN RM
Community Midwife, Devon, UK

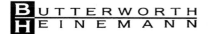

BUTTERWORTH
HEINEMANN

OXFORD AUCKLAND BOSTON JOHANNESBURG MELBOURNE NEW DELHI

Butterworth-Heinemann
Linacre House, Jordan Hill, Oxford OX2 8DP
225 Wildwood Avenue, Woburn, MA 01801-2041
A division of Reed Educational and Professional Publishing Ltd

A member of the Reed Elsevier plc group

First published 2000

© Reed Educational and Professional Publishing Ltd 2000

British Library Cataloguing in Publication Data
A catalogue record for this book is available from the British Library

Library of Congress Cataloguing in Publication Data
A catalogue record for this book is available from the Library of Congress

ISBN 0 7506 4378 1

Typeset by Bath Typesetting
Printed and bound by MPG Books Ltd, Bodmin, Cornwall

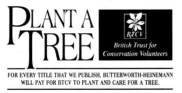

PLANT A TREE

BTCV
British Trust for
Conservation Volunteers

FOR EVERY TITLE THAT WE PUBLISH, BUTTERWORTH-HEINEMANN
WILL PAY FOR BTCV TO PLANT AND CARE FOR A TREE.

Contents

Foreword

I remember as a pre-clinical medical student, being told by a learned physiologist that 'one is more likely to die on the first day of life than on any other day except the last'. This of course still holds true but in the developed world, thanks to improving health, socio-economic status and obstetric care, the number of babies dying at or around birth has steadily fallen. However, we should never become complacent and as the 4th Confidential Enquiry into Stillbirths and Deaths in Infancy (CESDI) report indicates, babies are still lost as a direct consequence of inadequate resuscitation.

We live in changing times and the old medical training methods of 'see one, do one, teach one' are inadequate and unacceptable today. This is acutely focused during resuscitation where inexperience and unfamiliarity can and does lead to a worse outcome. Therefore, it behoves all health care professionals involved in the delivery of newborn babies to be familiar with and confident in the basic principles of neonatal resuscitation. The role of resuscitator is not exclusively medical and currently Advanced Neonatal Nurse Practitioners and Midwives regularly perform this task. As more professionals become responsible for resuscitation, the need for clear, unambiguous guidelines is crucial.

The authors have many years experience organizing and running resuscitation courses and this excellent book is a product of, and a tribute to, their success and hard work. This book admirably fills the gap between brief handbook and weighty textbook. The text is clear and well researched, the chapters follow a logical progression and the learning objectives of each chapter are clearly defined. Repetition of the systematic approach to resuscitation drives the key points home. As Professor Anthony Milner stated in 1991 'There can be few areas of medicine in which the potential benefit is so great but which have been subjected to so little evaluation.' In response to this, the emphasis is always placed on consensus of opinion and where there is a lack of consensus or clarity, a pragmatic approach is always taken. The difficult but important subject of when to stop and also when not to initiate resuscitation is dealt with in Chapter 16. I would urge readers to review this carefully and also become familiar with local guidelines and practices particularly at the limits of viability. Books on practical subjects will always have their limitations and this is freely acknowledged in this book. The importance of practice and maintenance of skills cannot be overemphasized and the authors make clear from the start, the need for resuscitation courses, regular training sessions and clinical exposure. As a basic text and supplement to these requirements I can wholeheartedly recommend this book to anyone involved in the care of newborn babies.

Dr Andrew Ewer MD MB ChB MRCP FRCPCH
Consultant Neonatologist
Birmingham Women's Hospital

Preface

Socioeconomic trends in the Western world and modern obstetric practice have benignly conspired to produce babies who are, in general, in increasingly better condition at birth. At the same time recent renewed interest in the practical and training aspects of neonatal resuscitation means that we are probably better equipped than ever before to cope with babies born in poor condition.

Nevertheless there remains an ever present need for the reappraisal and improvement of our practice. 'Care following delivery, mainly involving sub-optimal resuscitation of the newborn, was criticised in 81 of the 375 (22%) intrapartum related neonatal deaths' (CESDI, 1997).

That gentle cynic Qoheleth complained that even in his pre-print days 'to the making of many books there is no end'. We partly justify this contribution on the grounds that there are in fact few comprehensive treatments of the subject outside of larger textbooks.

We do recognize that neonatal resuscitation is a practical discipline and that this book can give no more than a theoretical background. In our opinion actual practice is best learned by a combination of the increasingly available Neonatal Advanced Life Support Courses and in-service training in the delivery suite. This book may help to prepare for this training but cannot replace it.

D. Drew
P. Jevon
M. Raby

Reference

Confidential Enquiry into Stillbirths and Deaths in Infancy (1997) *4th Annual Report*. Maternal & Child Health Consortium, London.

Acknowledgements

The authors would like to thank: the European Resuscitation Council for permission to reproduce their Resuscitation at Birth Flowcharts; John Hamilton and Anthea Insular, Medical Photography, Manor Hospital, Walsall for help with photographs; Wayne Smith, Medical Graphics and Jason McIntyre, Information Analyst, Manor Hospital, Walsall for help and advice with illustrations; Sharron Worth RGN LLB(Hons) Trainee Solicitor, Mills and Reeve for her assistance with writing the chapter 'Ethical and Legal Issues'.

Chapter 1

Adaptive changes at birth

Introduction

Most newborn babies breathe (cry even) spontaneously and establish an effective circulation more or less immediately at birth. A series of complex physiological changes, especially in the respiratory and cardiovascular systems, is necessary for this, usually, smooth transition from intrauterine to extrauterine life. This chapter describes in some detail these adaptive changes as a theoretical basis for resuscitation.

Chapter objectives

At the end of the chapter the reader will be able to:

- describe the circulation in fetal life
- outline the development of the fetal respiratory system
- describe sequentially the changes which take place in the respiratory and cardiovascular systems at birth.

The fetal circulation

The fetal circulation is complexly different to that of postnatal life (Fig. 1.1). Blood oxygenated in the placenta reaches the fetus by the umbilical vein. About half of this perfuses the liver and half enters the inferior vena cava by the ductus venosus. This mixes with the venous return from the liver and the lower half of the body and reaches the right atrium by the inferior vena cava.

Streaming within the right atrium results in this blood crossing to the left atrium by the foramen ovale. This blood is more highly oxygenated than blood returning by the superior vena cava and

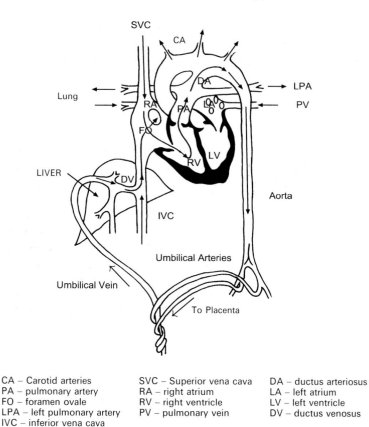

CA – Carotid arteries   SVC – Superior vena cava   DA – ductus arteriosus
PA – pulmonary artery   RA – right atrium   LA – left atrium
FO – foramen ovale   RV – right ventricle   LV – left ventricle
LPA – left pulmonary artery   PV – pulmonary vein   DV – ductus venosus
IVC – inferior vena cava

Fig. 1.1   Fetal circulation

constitutes the left ventricular output supplying the first part of the aorta. The coronary and carotid arteries in this way receive the most highly oxygenated blood available.

Blood returning to the right atrium by the superior vena cava largely flows into the right ventricle. A fraction of the right ventricular output enters the pulmonary circulation, but most of it passes through the ductus arteriosus into the arch of the aorta. The pulmonary circulation is maintained in a state of high vascular resistance during fetal life by a number of factors including relative hypoxaemia, mechanical factors, etc. The systemic circulation, on the other hand, is in a state of low resistance, largely because of the capacious placental vasculature. The pressure gradient this creates maintains the high level of right to left shunting across the ductus arteriosus routing less well oxygenated blood to the distal aorta. This supplies the lower parts of the body but the majority returns to the placenta by the umbilical arteries for re-oxygenation.

The fetal respiratory system

Prior to birth gas exchange is effected by the placenta and oxygenated blood supplied to the fetus by this specially adapted circulation. The lungs are full of lung fluid (about 30 ml/ kg body weight), which is a chloride-rich transudate from the lung capillaries. From about 16 weeks' gestation small amplitude fetal breathing movements are present (Lancet, 1989). These provide the mechanical stimulus for normal lung growth and development. In oligohydramnios, for example, where breathing movements are hampered by chest splinting, the lungs may become hypoplastic, i.e. underdeveloped.

Compared to postnatal life the lungs are underperfused, only about 10% of the blood leaving the right heart actually passing through the pulmonary circulation

Changes at birth

At birth most babies will breathe within the first minute. Exactly how this happens is still imperfectly understood but within a short time:

- the lungs will be fully expanded
- a functional residual capacity will have been established
- the lung fluid will be draining away
- the pulmonary and systemic circulations will be working in parallel, with shunting through the duct and foramen ovale having largely ceased.

The first breath

At birth the elastic recoil of the thorax draws air into the upper airway. The first breath is stimulated largely by hypoxaemia. Initially the lungs resist inflation because of the surface tension produced by fluid in the collapsed alveoli. Consequently high negative intrathoracic pressures are required to expand the lungs in the first instance.

Surfactant, produced by type 2 cells in the alveoli, stabilizes the alveoli once they have been inflated and prevents their collapse at the end of expiration. Surfactant production is fully established by about 32 weeks' gestation, but can be compromised by cold stress, hypoxia and acidosis, etc.

The lung fluid has partly (about one third) drained away during a normal vaginal delivery. The remainder will be actively removed by pumping sodium and hence water through ion channels in the alveolar endothelium into the pulmonary lymphatics. These channels open up in response to alveolar expansion and are modulated by catecholamines produced in labour. Failure to reabsorb lung fluid, especially common after elective caesarian section, produces a benign form of respiratory distress known as transient tachypnoea of the newborn (TTN).

Circulatory changes in the newborn

These changes in the respiratory system oxygenate the pulmonary vascular bed. In tandem with a number of other changes affecting smooth muscle tone in the pulmonary circulation, this produces a fall in pulmonary vascular resistance.

At the same time as the cord is cut and, with the exclusion of the placental circulation, systemic vascular resistance rises. This has the effect of increasing blood flow to the lungs and with the fall in the pressure gradient between the right and left side of the heart, the foramen ovale and the ductus arteriosus cease to shunt blood from right to left.

The systolic pressure in the aorta now actually exceeds that in the pulmonary artery and left to right shunting with oxygenated blood may occur. This is instrumental in causing duct closure. Evidence of this shunting can be heard in many healthy newborns in the first 12 hours of life in the form of a systolic murmur in the pulmonary area.

Chapter summary

An outline account has been given of the main changes in cardiovascular and respiratory function at and around the time of birth. Knowledge of these changes form an important basis for the practice of newborn resuscitation.

Chapter 2

Birth asphyxia and respiratory depression

Introduction

A small proportion of babies do not establish spontaneous effective breathing at birth. This is most commonly due to varying degrees of asphyxia, but may be due to other causes. Asphyxia is not easy to define. It is due to inadequate gas exchange causing hypoxaemia and a mixed acidosis from lactic acid production and carbon dioxide retention. Some of the clinical signs assessed by the Apgar score such as apnoea/bradypnoea, bradycardia, cyanosis and neurological impairment will be present depending on the severity of the asphyxia.

Chapter objectives

At the end of the chapter the reader will be able to:

- list the causes of respiratory depression at birth
- explain the normal phenomenon of intrapartum hypoxia and describe the fetal protective responses
- describe the sequence of pathophysiology in asphyxia as it relates to newborn resuscitation.

Causes of respiratory depression at birth

Respiratory depression at birth may occur for a number of reasons:

- intrapartum asphyxia
- drugs – narcotic analgesics, anaesthetics
- sepsis
- prematurity – CNS immaturity, surfactant deficiency, etc.
- respiratory problems – diaphragmatic hernia, obstructive lesions, etc.

- CNS abnormalities – malformations, trauma
- muscle disorders – myopathy, prematurity.

Intrapartum asphyxia is by far the commonest cause of respiratory depression at birth, but the above problems should also be considered during resuscitation. The general principles of resuscitation apply in each case, but there may be a need for specific interventions in individual conditions. These will be touched on in later chapters.

Intrapartum hypoxia and normal protective mechanisms

A degree of hypoxia is normal at birth. Typical umbilical artery blood gas values at delivery are as follows:

- pH 7.26
- Base deficit −7.8 mmol/l
- P_aCO_2 6.9 kPa
- P_aO_2 2.4 kPa.

This is transient hypoxia and is well tolerated by the neonate because of a remarkable capacity to minimize oxygen consumption while, at the same time, ensuring that vital organ systems are adequately perfused. The main mechanisms acting to protect the fetus during intrapartum hypoxia are as follows:

- the coronary and cerebral circulations are selectively provided with the most highly oxygenated blood by the specially adapted fetal circulation
- perfusion of the brain, heart and adrenal glands is maintained by selective vasoconstriction in non-essential organ systems
- heart muscle in particular has huge glycogen stores which provide substrate for anaerobic glycolysis to fuel myocardial contractions. This enables the heart to maintain an adequate output in the presence of hypoxia. It is only as profound acidosis develops that output is affected
- the normal response to hypoxia in the fetus, particularly in the last trimester, is slowing of the heart rate. This, with selective organ perfusion outlined above, minimizes energy and oxygen consumption
- the brain also has a number of mechanisms, which make it, at this period, exceptionally resistant to the effects of hypoxia. It too has rich glycogen stores and is capable of anaerobic glycolysis.

During hypoxia EEG changes indicate a shut down of energy-dependent processes. Even within the brain, preferential blood flow to the brain stem can occur to ensure that function in vital centres is maintained.

These mechanisms will continue to protect vital organs and even parts of organs during hypoxia. The human fetus is much more resistant to the effects of hypoxia than its adult counterpart. Although this cannot be exactly quantified, in rats for example, the fetus may be up to thirty times more resistant to hypoxia (Duffy *et al.*, 1975). After a certain duration of hypoxia which may vary with individual factors, such as gestation, intrauterine growth retardation coexisting chronic hypoxia, and other metabolic indices, these mechanisms are over-whelmed and cellular metabolism can no longer be maintained. In the later stages of this process organ systems including the brain, heart, lungs, kidneys and gut will become damaged, at first reversibly and then irreversibly so. Ultimately death ensues.

The pathophysiology of asphyxia

Much of what is known about the response to acute asphyxia in the fetus and newborn is derived from animal studies (Dawes, 1968). With certain reservations these have provided a clear insight into the process in humans and hence a logical basis for neonatal resuscitation. The interruption of an oxygenated blood supply via the umbilical vein may occur antepartum, intrapartum and will of course occur postpartum when the umbilical cord is cut. This is followed by a fairly predictable course of events as asphyxia becomes more severe (Fig. 2.1):

1. Initially there are a few breaths. These are intended to cause lung inflation, but if this occurs with the head in the birth canal, or if for one reason or another the lungs do not expand, this brief period of activity is followed by the complete cessation of breathing. This is known as *primary apnoea*.
2. After a short period, the length of which is not tested in the clinical situation since appropriate resuscitation measures are applied, automatic gasping starts. This is vigorous for a short time and then if the lungs are not inflated gradually declines in both force and frequency. The baby then enters a period of *terminal apnoea*. Unless vigorous resuscitation is commenced there will be no recovery from this terminal state.

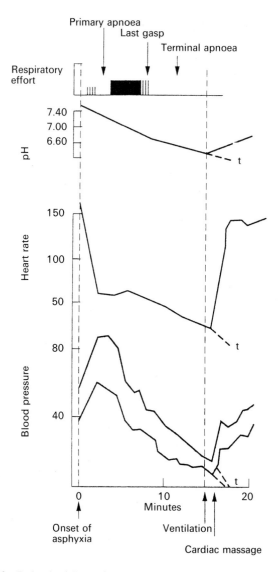

Fig. 2.1 Pathophysiology of asphyxia. (Adapted from Dawes *et al.*, 1963)

3. The heart rate falls throughout primary apnoea and eventually falls below 100 which is an internationally recognized action point in resuscitation – see chart 1, page 12.

There may be a small increase in heart rate during gasping but with its decline and end it continues to fall. As the acid–base state continues to deteriorate cellular metabolism fails and the heart stops. This may take a considerable time to happen.

4. During primary apnoea the blood pressure rises with the release of catecholamines and other stress chemicals. During terminal apnoea, however, it falls relentlessly in a close relationship with heart rate. Stroke volume is fixed in the neonate and cardiac output is determined almost entirely by heart rate.

5. From the onset of asphyxia there is an almost linear fall in pH. This is due to the accumulation of lactic and other acids produced by anaerobic glycolysis in hypoxic tissues. There is, however, unfortunately, a poor correlation between umbilical artery pH and immediate clinical state and long-term prognosis. In one recent study, no baby with a pH > 7.00 had any recognizable asphyxial complications. Of 23 babies with a pH < 7.00 only two had any such complications and these were babies recognizable clinically because of persistent low Apgar scores (Winkler *et al.*, 1991).

It may not always be possible to distinguish between primary and terminal apnoea. In general, profound bradycardia and the presence of shock are in favour of terminal apnoea. From the point of view of the resuscitation guidelines it is not necessary to make this distinction, actions being determined by the presence and degree of bradycardia.

Once effective resuscitation is begun, provided hypoxia and acidosis have not been too profound, there will usually be a rapid rise in heart rate and a gradual improvement in the metabolic part of the acidosis. In more severe hypoxia, where chest compressions are needed, there will be, in a successful resuscitation, a more gradual improvement in these parameters. When regular independent breathing starts will depend on the cause of the asphyxia, the severity of the asphyxia and the presence of any coexisting conditions such as prematurity, sepsis, etc.

Chapter summary

The causes of respiratory depression at birth resulting in the need for resuscitation have been outlined. The principal cause is intrapartum asphyxia. The pathophysiology of asphyxia and fetal protective mechanisms have been discussed.

Chapter 3

Resuscitation of the newborn – an overview

Introduction

The last 40 years have seen considerable improvements in the practice of newborn resuscitation. In theory at least, all babies should now be born in circumstances, whether in hospital or at home, where the facilities and expertise for resuscitation are available.

The principal aim of any resuscitation is to deliver healthy, breathing, pink babies to their parents or, where this is not possible, to ensure that babies, who are more seriously asphyxiated, are delivered to the neonatal unit in as good condition as is possible. This is achieved by a team effort with parental involvement, using methods and techniques about which there is widespread consensus. Following the publication of national and international guidelines (Royal College of Paediatrics and Child Health, 1997; European Resuscitation Council, 1998), all newborn resuscitation should follow the same logical and systematic approach. The purpose of this chapter is to provide an overview of this.

Chapter objectives

At the end of the chapter the reader will be able to:

- state the key objectives of resuscitation
- outline the required preparation
- outline the sequence of resuscitation of the newborn
- outline the importance of communication and documentation.

Objectives of resuscitation

The main objectives of resuscitation are to:

- minimize heat loss

- maintain a clear airway
- support breathing
- support circulation.

Preparation (see Chapter 4)

Current obstetric and midwifery practice has reduced the numbers of babies born in poor condition. Mechanical birth trauma is almost a thing of the past and CNS depression due to maternal analgesia and anaesthetics is uncommon.

Nevertheless, many cases of respiratory depression at birth still occur and wherever deliveries are taking place it is necessary to be fully prepared for resuscitation. Distress in some babies can sometimes be anticipated and provision made to ensure advanced help is immediately available. Preparation includes:

- anticipating the need to resuscitate
- ensuring an optimal thermal environment
- provision of resuscitation equipment
- staff training.

Minimizing heat loss and preventing the effects of cold stress is particularly important and will be emphasized throughout the text. Staff training will be discussed at length in Chapter 17.

Resuscitation sequence – The European Resuscitation Council Guidelines (ERC) for Resuscitation of Babies at Birth (1998) (see Chapters 4–10)

Resuscitation of a newborn baby should follow a systematic approach. This involves basic resuscitation first, progressing to advanced resuscitation only if the baby fails to improve. 'Time is of the utmost importance. Delay is damaging to the infant. Act promptly, accurately and gently' (Apgar, 1953). After half a century these recommendations still ring true.

The ERC guidelines (1998) incorporate two flow charts (Figs 3.1 and 3.2). Actions are prescribed for each specific situation. Once the action has been taken it is necessary to re-evaluate and take further action as appropriate until a stable situation has been reached. This is a simple but frequently neglected principle of resuscitation. It can be

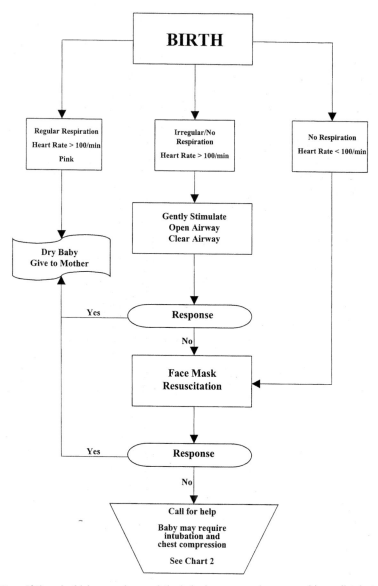

Note: If there is thick meconium and the baby is unresponsive, proceed immediately to Chart 2

Fig. 3.1 Resuscitation of the newborn chart 1

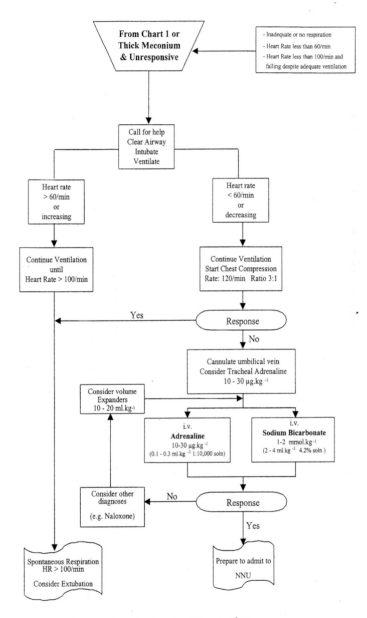

Note: Repeat adrenalin dose I.v. $100 \, \mu g.kg^{-1}$ if no response

Fig. 3.2 Resuscitation of the newborn chart 2

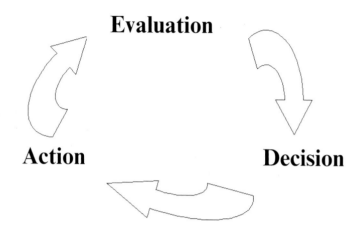

Fig. 3.3 Evaluation/decision/action cycle

represented by the Evaluation/Decision/Action Cycle (Fig. 3.3) and applies to all phases of the resuscitation.

The three key parameters which need to be evaluated are heart rate, respiratory activity and colour. Of these the heart rate is the most sensitive indicator of oxygenation. A rising heart rate indicates improved oxygenation, while a bradycardia or falling heart rate will suggest ineffective resuscitation. This constant re-evaluation is an integral part of the resuscitation process and is regularly emphasized throughout the text. It enables the practitioner to decide on the next appropriate action as recommended in the charts in Figures 3.1 and 3.2.

While birth asphyxia is the main reason for the newborn to need resuscitation, a number of other situations occur in the delivery room in which additional measures may be required. Some of these are described in detail in Chapter 11.

Post-resuscitation care (see Chapter 12)

All babies that have needed resuscitation require some initial monitoring, even if it is no more than recording vital signs and colour. Babies that are being transferred to the neonatal unit or another hospital, especially if oxygen-dependent or ventilated, will require electrical monitoring, e.g. oxygen saturation and heart rate. Chapter 12 discusses aspects of post-resuscitation management and transfer to definitive care.

Communication with parents

Where possible the parents should be seen before the delivery if problems are anticipated. They should be fully informed and involved at an appropriate level in decision making. Resuscitation takes priority until the baby is stable, but as soon as possible, someone who has been personally involved should speak to them. The importance of this is dealt with in Chapter 15, particularly in the context of bereavement, but good communication with parents must be recognized as an indispensable part of normal practice. This will be emphasized throughout the text.

Documentation and audit (see Chapter 14)

Full, detailed, sequential records must be kept for all resuscitations. Without this it is often difficult to make sense of what actually happened at the birth. These may also be of importance in any future medico-legal actions. In addition, they provide the material for audit whether it is the informal audit of the resuscitation process on the next ward round or a more formal audit of a series of resuscitations.

Resuscitation at home

Exactly the same sequence applies for resuscitation following home deliveries. Nevertheless, this situation presents a number of specific difficulties and these will be addressed in Chapter 13.

Chapter summary

This chapter has provided an overview of all the issues related to the resuscitation of the newborn.

Chapter 4

Preparing for resuscitation

Introduction

Being unprepared for a newborn resuscitation is probably the single factor most likely to prejudice a successful outcome. All resuscitations are stressful events and lack of preparation increases stress levels and may be a cause of conflict between professionals. Careful preparation needs to be made therefore. This involves advanced planning for the provision of an optimal environment for the newborn to minimize heat loss, adequate resources and equipment, and a high standard of training for resuscitators.

There should also be a locally agreed list of high-risk deliveries which should be attended by an experienced resuscitator. This will help minimize the risk of expert help not being immediately available to assist a distressed newborn.

Chapter objectives

At the end of the chapter the reader will be able to:

- discuss the importance of minimizing heat loss in the newborn baby and describe measures in the pre-delivery period to ensure an appropriate thermal environment
- list a minimal set of resuscitation equipment
- outline the roles of trained personnel
- list some of the high-risk deliveries which need to be attended by a skilled resuscitator
- outline the preparations required immediately prior to the delivery.

Minimizing heat loss

At birth the body temperature averages 37.8 °C, approximately one degree higher than the maternal temperature (Mann, 1968). However, the temperature can fall dramatically if measures are not taken to conserve heat. It is essential to avoid the metabolic complications of cold stress as even mild chilling may double oxygen requirements and significantly impair prospects for full recovery (Speidel *et al.*, 1998).

Measures should be taken both pre- and post-delivery and during any resuscitation attempt to minimize heat loss. Before discussing what steps can be taken in the pre-delivery period to minimize heat loss, at this stage, it will be helpful to outline why newborn babies are prone to heat loss, how they can lose heat and the effects of cold stress.

Why newborn babies have difficulty maintaining body temperature

All newborn babies, in particular the preterm and growth retarded, can have difficulty maintaining body temperature. Reasons for this include:

Heat losses in the newborn are high

- Large surface area compared with their body mass. Convective and radiant heat losses are increased particularly in a suboptimal thermal environment.
- Incomplete drying may lead to an increase in evaporative heat loss.
- Thin epidermis and a comparatively small amount of subcutaneous fat impairs insulation.

Newborns have limited ability to increase heat production

- Non-shivering thermogenesis from the breakdown of brown fat is the newborn's principal method of increasing heat production. In favourable conditions the heat production can be doubled (Hey, 1969), but even this may be insufficient to compensate for excessive losses.
- The non-shivering thermogenesis is limited in preterm and intrauterine growth-retarded babies who have poor fat stores.

In addition, any sick, hypoxic, acidotic or infected baby (i.e. those babies most likely to require resuscitation) will also have a limited ability to increase heat production.

How heat is lost

Heat can be lost in four different ways. This will determine the methods used to minimize heat loss.

- *Convection* – exposure in inadequately heated and draughty rooms.
- *Evaporation* – evaporation of water, e.g. from wet (amniotic fluid) skin. This is important in preterm babies because the immature skin offers little resistance to the diffusion of water. Water loss through the epidermis may be up to six times higher per unit surface area in a newborn of 26 weeks' gestation than in a term baby (Rutter and Hull, 1979).
- *Radiation* – radiation onto nearby solid objects.
- *Conduction* – to solid objects which the infant comes into contact with, e.g. an unwarmed cot mattress.

The adverse effects of heat loss

Excessive heat loss may cause or exacerbate:

- hypoxia (Stephenson *et al.*, 1970)
- metabolic acidosis (Gandy *et al.*, 1964) and delay recovery (Adamsons *et al.*, 1965)
- hypoglycaemia
- depletion of surfactant
- coagulatory disorders (Roberton, 1996).

Measures to minimize heat loss

There is usually some conflict of interest between the requirements of the labouring mother and the newborn. A compromise is best made by concentrating on the newborn's microenvironment, minimizing evaporative loss and applying radiant heat. Measures to minimize heat loss include:

- warm environment in the delivery room/theatre – 25 °C
- no draughts in the vicinity of the resuscitaire – windows closed

- warm dry towels immediately available
- warm resuscitation surface with radiant heater switched on.

The importance of minimizing heat loss during any resuscitation attempt and in the post-delivery period will be emphasized throughout the text.

Resuscitation equipment

All necessary resuscitation equipment should be immediately at hand and in working order. The following equipment should be available in the delivery room:

A warm, flat, slightly cushioned resuscitation surface with overhead radiant heat source and light; this will usually be a commercially-produced resuscitaire (Fig. 4.1).

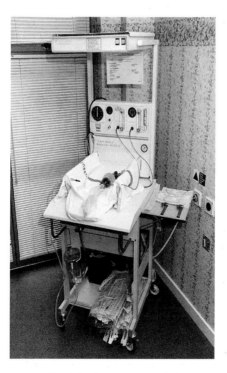

Fig. 4.1 Neonatal resuscitaire

Miscellaneous
  Gloves
  Apron
  Stop-clock
  Warm towels
  Stethoscope
  Scissors
  Tape
  Resuscitation flow charts.

Airway
  Suction source not exceeding minus 100 mmHg
  Suction catheters – sizes 6, 8 and 10 FG
  Oxygen/air supply with variable regulated flow rate and adjustable
    pressure relief valve
  Oxygen tubing
  Oropharyngeal airways, sizes 0 and 00
  Nasogastric tubes, sizes 5 and 8 FG.

Intubation
  Duplicate sets of laryngoscopes with blades 0 and 1; spare bulbs and
    batteries
  Tracheal tubes sizes 2.5, 3.0, 3.5 and 4.0 with adaptors
  Introducers
  Securing device.

Ventilation
  500 ml self-inflating resuscitation bag with oxygen reservoir or
    valved T-piece system
  Face masks sizes 0/0, 0/1
  Oxygen tubing.

Intravenous access
  Syringes and needles
  Sharps box
  Umbilical vein catheterization pack
  IV cannulae
  Pleural cannula set
  Intraosseous needle.

Medications/fluids
  Adrenaline 1 in 10 000 solution (100 μg/ml)
  Naloxone 400 μg/ml

Dextrose 10%
Sodium bicarbonate 4.2%
Volume expander 4.5% albumin
Sodium chloride 0.9%
Water for injection
Drug/fluid dosage chart.

Equipment inventory

- A complete inventory of equipment, should be available on the resuscitaire to facilitate regular checking.
- All resuscitaires should be identically stocked to avoid confusion.
- A system for daily documented checks of the inventory and that equipment is in working order should be in place. In addition, restocking after a resuscitation should be a specifically delegated responsibility.
- All mechanical equipment, e.g. resuscitaire, should be inspected and serviced on a regular basis by the electronics department following the manufacturer's recommendations.

Roles of trained personnel

Everyone with immediate responsibility for newborn care at delivery should have training in resuscitation. Chapter 17 deals with training issues at length. Traditionally junior and middle grade paediatricians have carried most of the responsibility, but both midwives and neonatal nurse practitioners are now playing an increasing role. Clear definition of responsibilities and roles within the team have to be determined locally.

Anticipating the need for resuscitation

There is a right balance between having highly trained paediatric staff intrusively present at every delivery and having those same doctors attend only when problems arise.

The former approach wastes valuable resources and medicalizes birth more than it is already and the latter puts babies at risk by potentially delaying resuscitation.

Identifying potentially high-risk deliveries and concentrating resources on these is part of the solution to this problem. Detailed below is a list of high-risk deliveries which can be used as a basis for local guidelines. They fall into three broad categories as recommended by the ERC (1998) with some overlap:

Delivery

Fetal distress
Reduced fetal movements before onset of labour
Abnormal presentation
Prolonged or difficult labour
Prolapsed cord
Prolonged rupture of membranes
Antepartum haemorrhage
Thick meconium-staining of liquor
Assisted deliveries
Emergency caesarean section.

Maternal

Severe pregnancy-induced hypertension
Heavy sedation
Drug addiction
Diabetes mellitus
Chronic illness
Concern of attending staff.

Fetal

Multiple pregnancy
Preterm, less than 34 weeks
Post-term, greater than 42 weeks
Growth restriction
Rhesus isoimmunization
Polyhydramnios
Oligohydramnios
Intrauterine infection.

Many so-called high-risk deliveries produce healthy screaming babies and even with modern technology some asphyxiated babies arrive without warning. Local audit may help to determine whether attendance at all of these deliveries is an effective use of resources.

Preparation immediately prior to delivery

There is a potential need for resuscitation with every delivery and consequently it is important to be always fully prepared. This involves the following:

- switch the resuscitaire light and heater on
- check that warm dry towels are available
- check all necessary equipment is available and in working order, in particular oxygen, suction, self-inflating bag and laryngoscopes
- wash hands and put on gloves.

In the event of a paediatrician being required, good communication with the obstetrician or midwife is vital. In an emergency call from the labour ward, a concise account of the details inasmuch as they are known is of great value. This may enable advice to be given over the phone and also may expediate the call for more senior help. In other less immediately urgent situations adequate time will be available for the paediatrician to go to the delivery room and personally clarify details with the obstetrician or midwife and read the notes if necessary. This may also provide an opportunity to meet the parents.

Chapter summary

The detailed preparations necessary to ensure optimal conditions for neonatal resuscitation have been described. These consist of a warm physical environment, provision of necessary equipment, training of personnel and the preparations that must be made for each delivery.

Chapter 5

Initial assessment at birth

Introduction

Chart 1 (Fig. 5.1) (ERC, 1998) is a simple flow chart for the initial evaluation and management of the newborn baby. Babies are divided into one of three groups on the basis of three simple clinical observations. Appropriate actions are prescribed for each of these three categories in turn. The vast majority of babies will need no more intervention than that outlined here.

Chapter objectives

At the end of the chapter the reader will be able to:

- describe the procedure immediately following birth
- describe a three-point clinical assessment used to assess babies
- use these three observations to classify all babies into one of three possible groups
- state appropriate actions to be taken in each case.

Procedure immediately following birth

- Start clock on resuscitaire at moment of delivery.
- Take baby in soft towelling and dry thoroughly. Discard wet towelling. Some mothers will have expressed their wish for the baby to be delivered directly onto their abdomen. This is a good heat source and provided the baby is vigorous will pose no problem.
- Most babies will be obviously crying, breathing and pinking up immediately following delivery. Apart from the most cursory

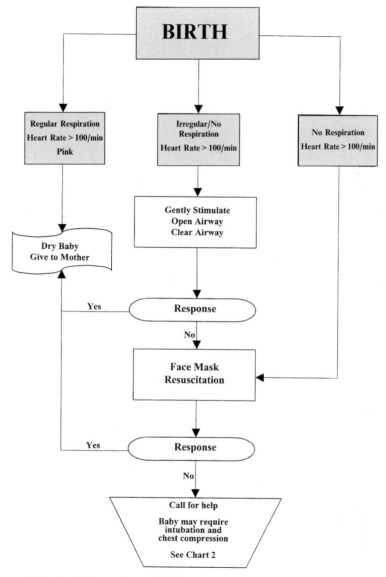

Note: If there is thick meconium and the baby is unresponsive, proceed immediately to Chart 2

Fig. 5.1 Resuscitation of the newborn chart 1

examination at this point do not delay in giving the baby to the mother (Fig. 5.2).

- Babies with thick meconium on the face at birth may be at risk of meconium aspiration. This is a special situation dealt with in Chapter 11.
- If not obviously breathing and vigorous place the baby supine on a flat surface (usually the resuscitaire mattress) under a radiant heater. Provided the baby has been dried properly, the overhead heater is on, the delivery room temperature is maintained at 25 degrees C and there are no draughts, it is not necessary to cover at this stage. Wrapping will hamper the immediate assessment and resuscitation (Fig. 5.3).

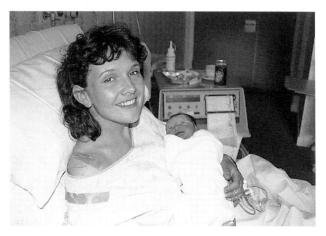

Fig. 5.2   Baby with mother

Three-point clinical assessment

A simple three-point assessment is now performed. This can easily be completed in 20 seconds.

Breathing

Carefully observe chest movement and air entry. If necessary auscultate. Also look for abnormal breathing patterns, e.g. asymmetrical chest movement, gasping or grunting.

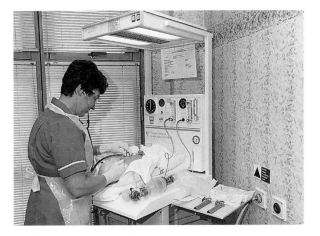

Fig. 5.3 Three-point assessment

Decide whether the breathing is *adequate* (good rate and regular), *inadequate* (slow and irregular) or *absent* altogether.

Heart rate

Estimate the heart rate either by auscultating the apex beat or feeling the umbilical pulsation.

Classify into > 100 or < 100 bpm (beats per minute). This is the accepted cut-off point indicating the presence or absence of significant hypoxia. *NB:* babies with a heart rate <*60* and especially babies with *no heart rate* will of course need a much more urgent approach. In the former, cardiac output may not, and in the latter definitely will not, even if ventilated, adequately perfuse the coronary arteries.

Colour

Check the lips and tongue which may be blue or pink. Peripheral cyanosis (acrocyanosis) is the norm in the first few hours and even days. A pale baby is likely to be shocked or possibly very anaemic. Decide whether the baby is *pink, blue* or *pale*.

These three observations will be easily recognizable as components of the Apgar score (Table 5.1). The other two components are tone and response to stimulation. These simply reflect CNS depression in the asphyxiated newborn unless of course there is an unrelated neuromuscular abnormality present.

Table 5.1 Apgar score chart

Score	0	1	2
Heart rate	Absent	< 100 b.p.m.	> 100 b.p.m
Respiratory effort	Absent	Irregular, slow	Regular, cry
Muscle tone	Limp	Some flexion in limbs	Well-flexed limbs
Reflex irritability	Nil	Grimace	Cough/cry
Colour	White	Blue	Pink

For many years Apgar scores have been recorded in a fairly mindless fashion without much notice being taken of how a particular score has been arrived at. This serves no purpose either in resuscitation or for long-term neurological prognosis. An assessment of breathing, heart rate and colour are all that are immediately required to guide the resuscitation. An Apgar score recorded at 10 minutes may be of some use for predicting prognosis.

Classification following clinical assessment

On the basis of these three observations any baby can be classified into one of the three following groups. Remember, however, that babies can quickly change groups, often for the worse, hence the need for frequent re-evaluation of these parameters.

Group 1

Adequate respiration
Heart rate > 100
Pink or improving.

The majority of newborn babies fall into this group. Often the situation will be clear even before the baby has been fully assessed. Give baby to mother.

Group 2

Inadequate or absent respiration
Heart rate > 100
Usually blue.

Ensure the airway is open and clear and gently stimulate. Administer 100% oxygen through a soft funnel mask. Visual monitoring of breathing and colour and tactile monitoring of the umbilical pulse can be maintained while this is being done. If the baby improves, moving into group 1, give baby to mother. If there is no improvement after a minute, earlier if despite these measures the pulse rate falls, start lung inflations. Babies responding to inflations but failing to breathe properly subsequently should be given naloxone if opiates have been given in the last 4 hours. Again, if the baby moves into category 1 continue as above. Normally if the baby is going to respond to these measures this will happen after the first 30 seconds or so of inflations. Failure to respond means the baby requires advanced life support. If a doctor with advanced resuscitation skills is not already present or has not been called this should now be done.

Group 3

No respiration
Heart rate < 100
Blue or white.

This represents a group of babies with various degrees of asphyxia. As with category 2 babies make sure the airway is open and clear. Give five lung inflations. Check that the lungs are expanding. If the heart rate is < 60 or < 100 and falling after these first inflations start chest compressions immediately. The guidelines (although not the texts) of the ERC and RCPCH may suggest that intubation must be performed before chest compressions are started. This needs some consideration. If lung inflation by face mask ventilation is effective and intubation likely to delay things by more than a few seconds continue with face mask ventilation. Specific indications for intubation are listed in Chapter 8.

A baby with a heart rate of 60 to 100 is just about as likely as babies in category 2 to respond to face mask ventilation. Again naloxone may be required if opiates have been used recently. Babies that make a rapid response may move straight into category 1. Observe on resuscitaire for a while. Give to the mother when settled, pink and breathing regularly.

A few babies with bradycardia do not respond to lung inflation and will continue to deteriorate unless appropriate action is taken. The commonest reason for this is ineffective inflation usually due to poor technique. Those that need compressions from the start and babies not responding to inflations, with the heart rate falling, are now in need of advanced life support.

Chapter summary

The procedure for initial assessment and care of the newborn immediately following delivery has been outlined. This consists of simple measures applicable to all newborn and a logical scheme of clinical assessment and application of the results of this to a flow chart to determine appropriate actions.

Chapter 6

Open and clear airway, gently stimulate

Introduction

The Group 2 baby is not breathing at all or breathing inadequately and cyanosed, but the hypoxia is of an insufficient severity to have caused bradycardia. This situation needs resuscitatory measures which, though simple, need to be done properly. These include the initial drying and warming, airway opening and clearing techniques which are done prior to the assessment. This is followed in this group of mildly depressed babies by mechanical stimulation if there is no sign of improvement and the administration of facial oxygen (Fig. 6.1).

Chapter objectives

At the end of this chapter the reader will be able to:

- describe the methods of airway opening which will most facilitate resuscitation
- describe methods of airway suction and their possible adverse consequences
- describe recommended methods of mechanical stimulation and some of the dangers
- state the indication for administering facial oxygen.

Airway opening

Place the baby supine on a flat, firm surface, preferably a resuscitaire. Some resuscitaires still retain the ability to raise the foot end. This puts an extra load on the diaphragm and increases the work of breathing. In babies with congenital ascites it may be an advantage to position

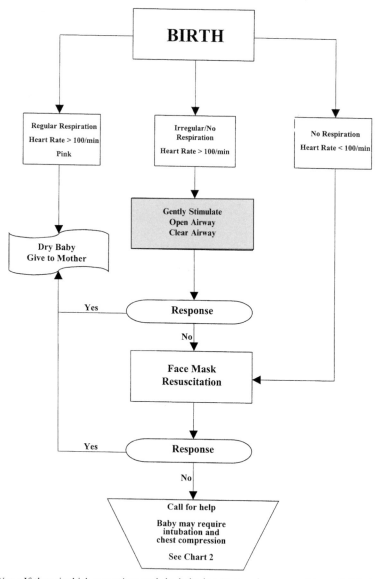

Note: If there is thick meconium and the baby is unresponsive, proceed immediately to Chart 2

Fig. 6.1 Resuscitation of the newborn chart 1

foot down until fluid has been removed.

Babies have a large occiput and on a flat surface fall naturally into a position of neck flexion (Fig. 6.2c).

The position for optimal airway opening is called the neutral position. This is best achieved with a small towel placed under the shoulders (Fig. 6.2a). Over-extension of the neck may occur if the head is allowed to drop over the end of the mattress or if excessive head-tilt is applied (Fig. 6.2b).

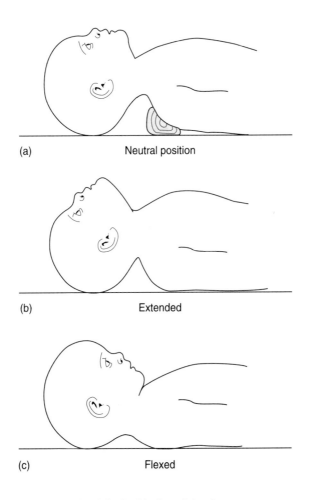

(a)   Neutral position

(b)   Extended

(c)   Flexed

Fig. 6.2 Positioning of the airway

Once in the neutral position lift the chin slightly with one finger to prevent the tongue causing obstruction. Take care to apply the finger to the point of the chin and not the soft-tissues below the jaw as this will cause obstruction.

Airway suction

Most babies require no airway clearance. If there are obvious quantities of meconium, blood, etc. in the airway it should be aspirated. If there is obvious respiratory effort but no chest expansion, suck out the airway. This is best undertaken with an electronic suction device with a vacuum not exceeding minus 100 mmHg. Use a 10 FG catheter (8 FG in a preterm) and suction out the pharynx first and then, if necessary, the nose. This will help avoid aspiration if nasal suction provokes a gasp. In the event of thick meconium being present suck out under direct vision with a laryngoscope (see Chapter 11).

Avoid deep, blind, prolonged suction. This may produce reflex apnoea, vagally-induced bradycardia and make the existing hypoxia worse (Codero and How, 1971). Even with soft catheters it is still possible to traumatize the delicate mucosa especially in the premature. So take care. It is recommended that the catheter tip should not be inserted further than 5 cm. In addition, each suction attempt should not last longer than 5 seconds (Royal College of Pediatrics and Child Health, 1997). Ideally the heart rate should be continually monitored by an assistant.

Drying, airway opening and any suction will have helped stimulate respiratory activity and this may be quite obvious on re-evaluation. An improving, pink and vigorous baby can be passed to the mother. If there is no response it will now be appropriate to stimulate with the specific objective of improving breathing.

Tactile stimulation

A number of different methods are described. A single finger flick to the sole of the foot will give an indication as to whether tactile stimulation is likely to be effective (Fig. 6.3). If so it is likely to produce facial grimacing, an obvious increase in respiratory effort or even a cry. How hard to flick is a matter of judgement, but it is important not to cause significant pain and under no circumstances should it cause bruising. Another safe method is gentle rubbing of the back. A number of unsafe methods of stimulation have been used including back slapping and sternal pressure. These may cause injury and should not be used.

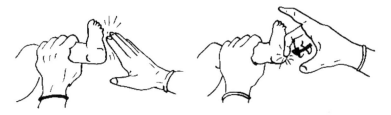

Fig. 6.3 Flicking the feet

Oxygen

Babies who are breathing inadequately and cyanosed should receive facial oxygen by a soft funnel (Figure 6.4).

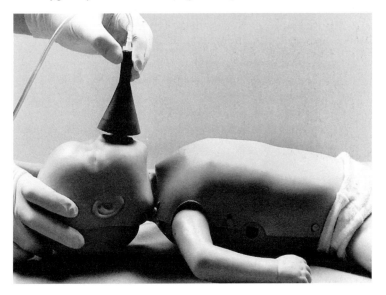

Fig. 6.4 Administration of oxygen via a soft funnel

This will probably speed up recovery from hypoxia. Giving facial oxygen to an apnoeic baby serves little purpose unless perhaps it is administered during tactile stimulation which may provoke inspiration. Some babies appear to be breathing normally and yet remain cyanosed. These should receive oxygen but probably have either persistence of the fetal circulation or a cyanotic form of congenital heart disease.

Re-assessment of the baby

If the baby has established regular respirations and is pinking up hand her over to the mother. If the baby is still not breathing and has failed to respond to airway opening and clearing, gentle tactile stimulation and oxygen, face mask resuscitation is now indicated.

Chapter summary

Babies with mild hypoxia (inadequate respiration but heart rate > 100) have been described and may breathe spontaneously following the stimulation from routine drying and movement to the resuscitaire. Those who do not respond may do so following airway opening and clearance and a little additional stimulation and facial oxygen.

Chapter 7

Face mask resuscitation

Introduction

Face mask ventilation is the most commonly used method of inflating the newborn's lungs. It is effective and relatively safe in experienced hands. Besides inflating the lungs mechanically it probably also works by stimulating Head's paradoxical reflexes, i.e. the inflation pressure induces the baby to make respiratory efforts (Milner, 1998).

Chapter objectives

At the end of the chapter the reader will be able to:
- list the indications and contraindications for face mask ventilation
- list the equipment required
- describe two methods of face mask resuscitation
- list the possible causes of ineffective face mask ventilation.

Indications

- No or ineffective respiration despite airway opening and clearing, tactile stimulation and facial oxygen, with a falling heart rate (Fig. 7.1).
- No respiration and heart rate < 100 beats per minute.

Contraindications

- Meconium or other aspiration syndromes.
- Diaphragmatic hernia.

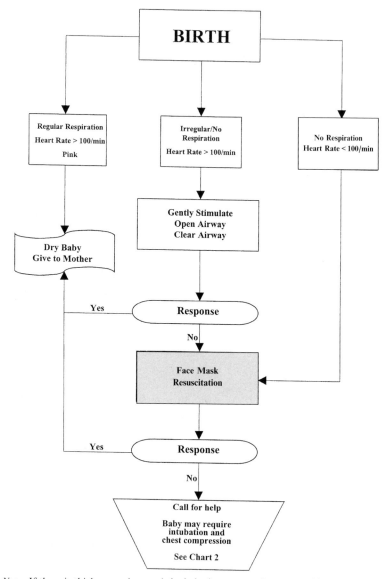

Note: If there is thick meconium and the baby is unresponsive, proceed immediately to Chart 2

Fig. 7.1 Resuscitation of the newborn chart 1

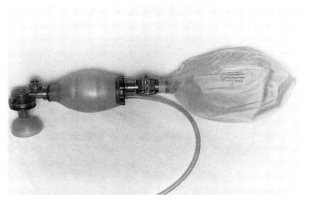

Fig. 7.2   Bag/valve/mask device

Methods

There are three methods of applying face mask resuscitation:

- self-inflating bag (often referred to as bag/valve/mask) (Fig. 7.2)
- valved T-piece
- anaesthetic bag.

In practice the self-inflating bag is by far the most popular method, though the valved T-piece has a number of advantages and may find increasing use in the future. Paediatricians and midwives rarely have any experience using the anaesthetic bag in the delivery room and therefore it will not be discussed further.

Self-inflating bag

The face mask

Face masks (Fig. 7.3) come in a variety of different shapes, sizes and materials. For newborn resuscitation the mask should have the following characteristics:

- circular shape (rigid triangular masks are not recommended as they are more prone to air leakage (Palme *et al.*, 1985)
- a soft cushioned rim that will conform to the contour of the

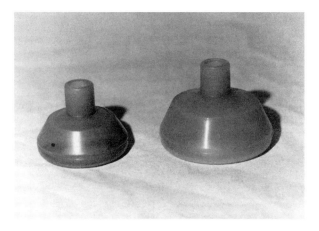

Fig. 7.3 Face masks

baby's face making it easier to form a seal, which is essential for effective lung inflation
- availability in a choice of sizes, usually 00 and 0/1
- made of transparent silicone so that secretions, etc. can be easily seen
- minimal dead space.

Choose an appropriate sized mask that will fit snugly over both mouth and nose but will neither cause pressure on the eyes or create an air leak by over-riding the chin.

The self-inflating bag

There are a number of different makes of self-inflating bag available, but they all work on the same principle. Personnel using this device ought to be familiar with its structure and function. The self-inflating bag (see Fig. 7.2) consists of the following components (Fig. 7.4):

- the bag (A)
- the air inlet (B)
- the oxygen inlet (C)
- oxygen reservoir bag (D)
- the patient outlet (E).

The valve system consists of four valves:

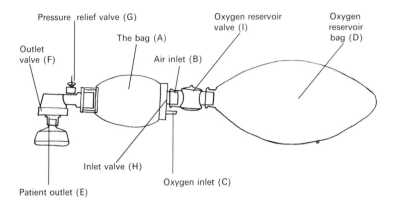

Fig. 7.4 Face masks: appropriate size and position

- the outlet valve between bag and mask or tube (F)
- the pressure relief valve (G)
- the inlet valve between bag and air inlet (H)
- the oxygen reservoir valve (I)

The bag (A) Different bag sizes are available. The 500-ml bag should be used for newborn resuscitation. It will reinflate by recoil after being squeezed even if no gas is entering.

The air inlet (B) Oxygen is sucked through the air inlet if the oxygen reservoir bag is full and attached. If it is not attached, air will be sucked through.

The oxygen inlet (C) Oxygen is delivered to the bag here at a recommended rate of 10 l/min (if the oxygen tubing is connected and the flowmeter turned on!).

The reservoir bag (D) With an oxygen flow rate of 10 l/min this will increase the oxygen concentration delivered to the baby to almost 100% (Laerdal, 1997). Oxygen is allowed to fill the reservoir during expiration enabling the rapid refilling of the bag.

The patient outlet (E) This connects directly to the face mask or the tracheal tube adapter.

The valve system These are practically the only parts of the apparatus that can malfunction, usually if they have been wrongly reassembled which, on most models, is now difficult to do. There are four valves.

The outlet valve (F) This is situated between the bag and patient outlet, it opens when the bag is squeezed allowing gas through to the baby.

The pressure relief valve (G) This is situated between the bag and outlet valve, it opens at about 30–40 cmH$_2$O preventing very high pressures being generated. The valve has rather low inertia but higher pressures can be generated with this device if an incorrect, jerky technique is used. Some valves have an over-ride clip for inflating very stiff lungs, but this must be used with caution, if at all, because of the risk of pneumothorax.

The inlet valve (H) This is situated between the bag and air inlet, it allows air to enter the bag during refilling but prevents exit during squeezing.

The oxygen reservoir valve (I) This allows excess oxygen to escape, therefore no problem with an oxygen flow rate of 10 l/min.

Procedure

1. Ensure the airway is open. Reposition and clear if necessary. The main skill in using the self-inflating bag effectively is keeping the airway open while delivering inflations.
2. Set the oxygen flow at 10 l/min and ensure the oxygen reservoir bag is expanding – this will deliver close to 100% oxygen (Laerdal, 1997).
   Alternatively 50% oxygen is sometimes used if gas mixing facilities are available (European Resuscitation Council, 1998). There is some evidence that resuscitation with air rather than 100% oxygen results in a more rapid recovery. However, there is no evidence that it improves Apgar scores or neurological status (Ramji *et al.*, 1993).
3. Choose an appropriate sized mask and position it on the face so that it covers the nose and mouth and ensure a good seal. Care should be taken not to apply pressure on the soft tissues under the jaw as this may obstruct the airway (Fig. 7.5).

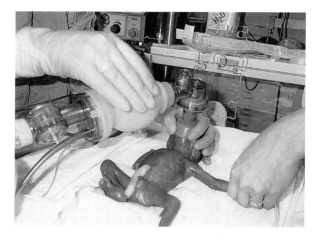

Fig. 7.5 Use of bag/valve/mask device

4. Deliver five sustained inflations. Each should ideally last 1–2 seconds. Prolonging these first inflations helps overcome the initial resistance to lung expansion and will help produce a functional residual capacity more quickly (Vyas *et al.*, 1981). Use a 500-ml bag as a smaller 250-ml bag does not permit sustained inflation. (In practice it can be difficult to maintain pressure for longer than 0.5 seconds with a 500-ml bag.) Higher pressure will be generated in these first inflations and special care is required to maintain the air-seal.

5. Look for chest movement. Ask an assistant to auscultate for breath sounds. Also look at and listen to the epigastrium for signs of the stomach inflating. A nasogastric tube can be inserted if this becomes a problem.

6. Ventilate at a rate of 30 breaths per minute. Note that some babies with heart rates < 60 and no immediate improvement will need chest compressions at this stage. This is not entirely clear on the ERC flow charts, which may appear to suggest that compressions should only be started if tracheal intubation has been performed.

   Compressions can be started before intubation provided that face mask ventilation is adequate. Intubation then becomes a priority. If tracheal intubation is likely to interrupt adequate ventilation by face mask more than momentarily (inexperienced operator or difficult intubation), it should be delayed until the baby is more stable or more experienced help is available.

7. If ventilation is judged ineffective recheck airway patency and the face mask seal. Consider equipment failure. In each case take appropriate action. If the lungs are known to be stiff, a higher inflation pressure can be tried by disabling the pressure relief valve, but intubation is a better option.

8. Continue to ventilate and reassess. If adequate spontaneous breathing starts, discontinue ventilation. Additional oxygen may be required by soft funnel mask. If narcotics have been given in the previous 4 hours and the onset of breathing is delayed beyond the baby becoming pink with a normal heart rate, give naloxone. Any baby who recovers quickly and fully after this level of resuscitation can go to the ward with the mother unless there is some other specific indication for admission to the neonatal unit.

9. Babies who do not breathe at this stage require intubation and possibly transfer to the neonatal unit for further management.

Face mask T-piece

This method of ventilation, a simple alternative to the self-inflating bag, was first described in 1926 and is currently the subject of renewed interest. It consists of a soft silicone mask as described above with an oxygen supply and a pressure relief valve similar to those built into most modern resuscitaires. A T-piece to interrupt oxygen delivery is incorporated at the mask end. A commercial system, the Neopuff (Fig. 7.6) is also available.

The procedure is similar to that used with the self-inflating bag. The pressure valve should be set at 30 cmH$_2$O for the first five breaths and inflation sustained for 2 seconds until the chest has expanded and then reduced to a pressure that produces good chest movement.

Advantages of face mask T-piece resuscitation

- Requires only one hand to operate, thus leaving the other hand free.
- The pressure control is more flexible.
- Facilitates the delivery of more sustained inflation pressures for initial lung expansion.
- Routine use may reduce the need for intubation by up to 50% (Milner, 1991).

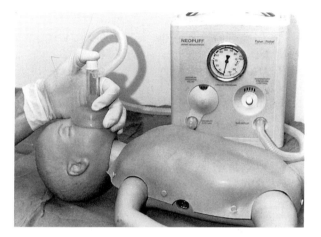

Fig. 7.6 The Neopuff

Chapter summary

Two methods of face mask ventilation have been described. The self-inflating bag is in near-universal use and is effective and safe with good technique. The equipment is described in some detail as doctors and midwives, even those who use it regularly, often do not understand how it works. Standard texts and guidelines do not usually give these details. The alternative method using a T-piece is less popular but may have some advantages.

Chapter 8

Tracheal intubation

Introduction

Too much emphasis may be placed on the skill of intubation which can lead to doctors and midwives lacking confidence in their ability to resuscitate unless they have mastered it.

Face mask resuscitation is quite adequate in most babies and wider use of the face mask with T-piece may bring the intubation rate down further. There is significant variation in intubation rates between different hospitals and it is hard to believe this is because in some the rate is too low.

Nevertheless, the advanced resuscitator must be able to intubate quickly and safely and the skill must be mastered and maintained. Reports with titles such as 'Traumatic vocal cord injury in a newborn' emphasize the dangers of the technique in unskilled hands.

Chapter objectives

At the end of the chapter the reader will be able to:
- state the indications for intubation
- list the equipment required
- describe the procedure for intubation
- discuss the post-intubation checks
- list the causes of ineffective ventilation following intubation and outline actions to be taken.

Indications for intubation (Fig. 8.1)

- Need for tracheal suction, e.g. aspirated blood or meconium.
- Ineffective face mask ventilation.

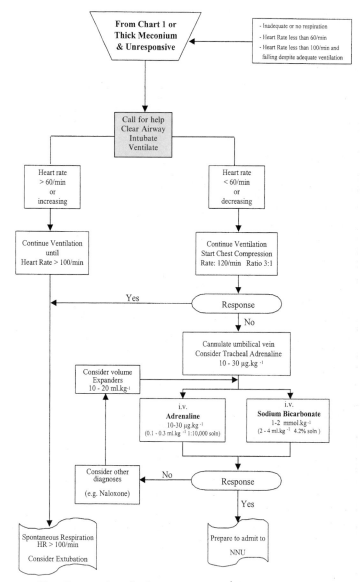

From Chart 1 or
Thick Meconium
& Unresponsive

- Inadequate or no respiration
- Heart Rate less than 60/min
- Heart Rate less than 100/min and
  falling despite adequate ventilation

Call for help
Clear Airway
Intubate
Ventilate

Heart rate
> 60/min
or
increasing

Heart rate
< 60/min
or
decreasing

Continue Ventilation
until
Heart Rate > 100/min

Continue Ventilation
Start Chest Compression
Rate: 120/min Ratio 3:1

Response   Yes

No

Cannulate umbilical vein
Consider Tracheal Adrenaline
10 - 30 µg.kg^{-1}

Consider volume
Expanders
10 - 20 ml.kg^{-1}

i.v.
Adrenaline
10-30 µg.kg^{-1}
(0.1 - 0.3 ml.kg^{-1} 1:10,000 soln)

i.v.
Sodium Bicarbonate
1-2 mmol.kg^{-1}
(2 - 4 ml.kg^{-1} 4.2% soln)

Consider other
diagnoses
(e.g. Naloxone)

No   Response

Yes

Spontaneous Respiration
HR > 100/min

Consider Extubation

Prepare to admit to
NNU

Note: Repeat adrenalin dose I.v. 100 µg.kg^{-1} if no response

Fig. 8.1 Resuscitation of the newborn chart 2

- Extreme prematurity and surfactant administration.
- Prolonged ventilation.
- Transfer.
- Diaphragmatic hernia.

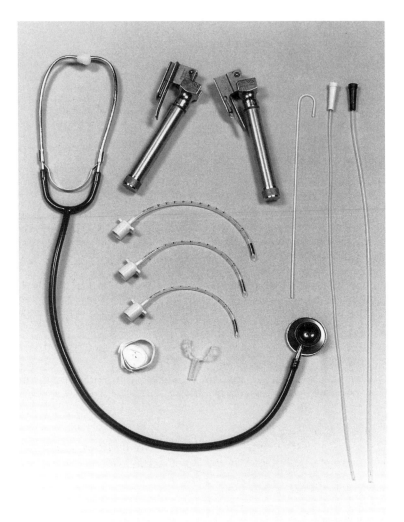

Fig. 8.2 Equipment for intubation

Equipment (Fig. 8.2)

- Two straight bladed laryngoscopes and spare (no. 0 and no. 1).
- Tracheal tubes – sizes 2.5, 3.0, 3.5 and 4.0.
- Flexible introducer.
- Suction apparatus and catheters.
- Oxygen supply.
- Self-inflating bag.
- Fixing materials.
- Stethoscope.

Some of this equipment will now be described in more detail.

Tracheal tube

Common characteristics

There are two main kinds of tracheal tube. Straight tubes (Fig. 8.3a) and shouldered tubes known as the Coles tube (Fig. 8.3b). The Coles tube is still used for resuscitation, but a straight tube with an introducer is the most popular. Most straight tubes have the following:

- a black area at the tip, the 'vocal cord guide'. This is the point up to which the tube should be inserted through the vocal cords. This usually results in the tube tip resting in the middle third of the trachea
- graduations (in centimetres) which, not only act as a guide during insertion, but also help detect tube slippage
- a standard 15 mm adapter which enables connection of the tube to the self-inflating bag or T-piece.

Tracheal tube size

This is graded by the internal tube diameter in millimetres. The correct size is normally determined by the weight of the baby.

Less than 1000 g	size 2.5
1000–2500 g	size 3.0
Greater than 2500 g	size 3.5

An alternative method of estimating the approximate correct size is by using gestational age:

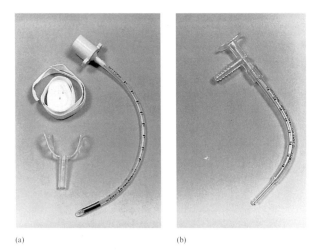

(a)   (b)

Fig. 8.3   Straight and Coles tubes

$$\text{Tube size} = \frac{\text{gestational age in weeks}}{10}$$

Whichever method is used, it must be remembered that this is only a guide and tubes one size smaller and one size larger should be immediately available. Size 2.0 ET tubes should not be used because their high resistance prevents effective ventilation.

Tracheal introducer

A tracheal tube introducer made of plastic-covered soft metal wire can facilitate intubation by increasing the stiffness of the tube and its curvature. Ensure that the introducer tip does not protrude beyond the end of the tube as this can cause soft tissue trauma. Bend the introducer back over the adapter to prevent it slipping down the tube.

Laryngoscope

- Use a straight bladed laryngoscope with a light-weight alloy handle for newborn intubation.
- Blade size 1 will be adequate for most babies, but size 0 may be required for larger babies.
- Ensure that the bulb is working and is not loose prior to the procedure.
- Have a spare, working, laryngoscope at hand.

Procedure for intubation

Preparation

1. Ensure all the equipment listed above is available and in working order.
2. Position the baby on a flat surface, preferably a resuscitaire, and extend the neck into the 'neutral position' (Fig. 8.4). A rolled up towel placed under the shoulders will help maintain proper alignment of the mouth, pharynx and trachea.

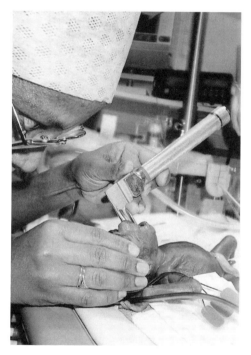

Fig. 8.4 Intubation–visualizing the vocal cords

3. Ensure the neck is not over-extended as this will lift the glottis out of the line of sight and also narrow the trachea. Similar difficulties in visualization and intubation will occur if the head is too flexed.
4. Pre-oxygenate for about 30 seconds if possible (i.e. if the lungs

will inflate with face mask resuscitation) and if safe to do so (i.e. no meconium, etc. in the airway). Ask an assistant to monitor the baby's heart rate during the procedure.

Visualizing the vocal cords

5. Hold the laryngoscope in the left hand (irrespective of handedness) while the right stabilizes the baby's head.
6. Gently insert the laryngoscope into the baby's mouth past the uvula until the epiglottis comes into view. At this point there are two possible methods for visualizing the vocal cords. This is a matter of personal preference. Either place the tip of the blade in the vallecula (a groove slightly anterior to the epiglottis) or override and capture the whole epiglottis.
7. Lift the laryngoscope upwards and forwards along the line of the handle. This will bring the vocal cords into view. If the laryngoscope has been inserted too far the oesophagus will be seen. If not far enough only the pharyngeal wall or tongue will be seen. It is essential to avoid lifting just the tip of the blade by using a rocking motion and pulling the handle towards the operator. This will fail to show the vocal cords and may damage the upper gum.
8. Gentle pressure on the cricoid cartilage, with the little finger of the left hand or by an assistant, will help to bring the vocal cords into view, but this is not usually needed if intubation technique is correct.
9. The cords can now be visualized. Suction if necessary.

Inserting the tracheal tube

10. Take the tube, preferably fitted with an introducer with a slight curve, in the right hand. Pass the tube down the right side of the blade in the direction of the cords which should be kept in view. Only advance the tube if it can be seen where it is being inserted; it is only likely to enter the trachea if it is visualized doing so.
11. Advance the tube through the cords until the black 'vocal cord guide' has passed through the cords.
12. If the vocal cords are in spasm wait a few seconds. Attempting to pass the tube through closed cords may damage them and exacerbate the spasm.

13. Connect to the self-inflating bag or valved oxygen supply.
14. Give five sustained inflations lasting about 2 seconds (or as long as practical up to 2 seconds).
15. Check that the lungs are inflating adequately. Look for bilateral chest movement and auscultate the chest. Good chest movement and air entry will usually on reassessment be followed by an increase in heart rate and an improvement in colour.

Ineffective ventilation following intubation

Ventilation may not be established effectively after intubation or, if it is, may become ineffective after a variable period. The main causes of this are described by the acronym DOPES:

- *D*isplaced tube. The tube may be displaced into the pharynx, oesophagus, right or left main bronchus.
- *O*bstructed tube. This is unusual initially unless meconium or pus etc. are present.
- *P*neumothorax.
- *E*quipment failure.
- *S*tiff lungs.

These problems should be recognized and diagnosed by the checks that routinely follow intubation (Table 8.1).

Securing the tube

Firmly secure the tube by the locally agreed method. The length of the tracheal tube at the lips should be noted as this will help to detect tube migration.

Possible complications of intubation

- Hypoxia. Pre-oxygenate before intubation where possible. If intubation is unsuccessful re-oxygenate after 30 seconds.
- Bradycardia/apnoea. This can be caused by hypoxia or by a vagal response induced by stimulation of the posterior pharynx by the laryngoscope blade, tracheal tube or suction catheter. Ensure that the baby's heart rate is monitored by an assistant during the procedure.

Table 8.1

Problem	Signs	Action
Displaced tracheal tube		
1. Oropharynx	No air entry to lungs Audible air leak Tube short at the mouth	Remove tube, pre-oxygenate if possible and re-intubate
2. Oesophagus	No air entry to the lungs Stomach inflating	Remove tube, pre-oxygenate if possible and re-intubate
3. Main bronchus	No air entry in opposite lung	Withdraw tube slowly, listening for breath sounds on the collapsed side
Obstructed tracheal tube	Resistance to inflation noted Consider stiff lungs	1. Try suction down the tube 2. If no change, remove tube and pre-oxygenate if possible and re-intubate
Pneumothorax (tension)	Reduced air entry over affected side Chest over inflated	Decompress the chest (see page 79)
Equipment	Unexplained deterioration or difficulty with resuscitation	Check oxygen supply Check equipment and replace if necessary
Stiff lungs	Poor chest expansion and air entry, this is normal with first inflations RDS in prematures	Increase pressure Surfactant therapy

- Soft tissue damage to the lips, pharynx, larynx, trachea, oesophagus, etc.

Chapter summary

Tracheal intubation has been described in the overall context of neonatal resuscitation. A basic equipment set has been listed and a detailed description of the method given. This must, nevertheless, be supplemented with practical training with manikins and in the labour ward. The post-intubation checks and possible problems remembered as DOPES are given.

Chapter 9

Chest compressions

Introduction

Asphyxia produces a complex set of metabolic changes consisting principally of tissue hypoxia, metabolic acidosis (lactic acid, etc. produced by anaerobic glycolysis) and respiratory acidosis (hypercapnia). As these become more severe they cause deterioration in organ function, most critically in the heart (see Chapter 2).

Initially, by selective vasoconstriction to non-essential organs, the blood supply to the heart and brain is preserved. As the heart rate continues to fall and with it, cardiac output, even circulation to these organs is compromised. In the earlier stages of this process oxygenation by effective lung inflation will restore the heart rate to normal.

In the later stages, however, with very low cardiac output, blood in the pulmonary circulation, which is being oxygenated by lung inflations, cannot physically reach the coronary circulation to relieve the myocardial hypoxia. In addition, circulation to the brain is failing with the attendant risk of hypoxic brain damage.

Chest compressions are an effective and accepted method in this situation for perfusing the coronary and cerebral circulations. Once the coronary circulation is re-established and the heart rate restored the rest of the systemic and the pulmonary circulation is likely to follow (Fig. 9.1).

Chapter objectives

At the end of this chapter the reader will be able to:

- list the indications for chest compressions
- describe two different methods of chest compression

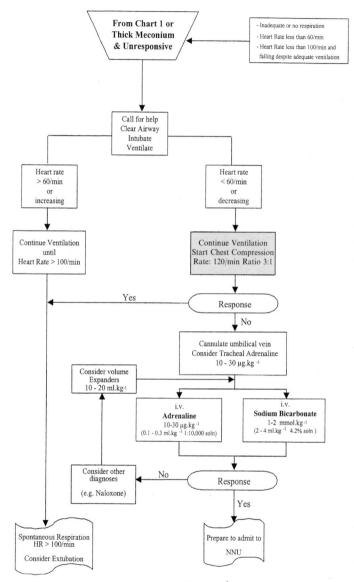

Note: Repeat adrenalin dose I.v. $100 \, \mu g.kg^{-1}$ if no response

Fig. 9.1 Resuscitation of the newborn chart 2

- critically compare these two methods
- describe the reassessment required following compressions
- list the indications for discontinuing compressions.

Indications

Chest compressions should be performed if the heart rate is:

- less than 60 or
- between 60 to 100 and falling despite adequate ventilation.

Methods

Compressions require an extra pair of hands, therefore summon help if not already available. There are two accepted methods for performing chest compressions known as the two-thumb method and the two-finger method respectively. The main principles of these methods are the same and are described as follows:

Landmarks

- Apply the fingers or thumbs over the lower third of the sternum, i.e. about one finger's breadth below the inter-nipple line (Phillips and Zideman, 1986). Compressions performed anywhere near the xiphoid process are likely to cause visceral damage, especially to the liver.

Rate

- 90 per minute. (We diverge from the ERC and RCPCH guidelines here.) In practice a rate of 120 compressions per minute (two per second) is difficult to achieve and almost impossible to sustain (Whyte *et al.*, 1998, 1999). The American Heart Association guidelines (1997) recommend 120 events per minute, i.e. 90 compressions and 30 inflations. Other authorities (Northern Neonatal Network, 1996) recommend even lower rates of compressions such as 40–60 per minute. These rates are not evidence-based. The aim of compressions is to perfuse the coronary circulation, not the whole body.

Ratio

- Three chest compressions to one ventilation (3:1), resulting in 90 compressions and 30 ventilations per minute as above.
- About 0.5 seconds is required for each inflation. This requires a pause in compressions. Exhalation takes place during compressions. In practice these rates and ratios are difficult to deliver with any precision and this probably is not too important.

Depth

- In a term baby the recommended compression depth is 2–3 cm, which is approximately one third of the anterior–posterior chest diameter.

Action

- The action should be well controlled, not be jerky or erratic, as this will increase the likelihood of trauma.
- ERC guidelines state that the chest wall should be allowed to return fully to its relaxed position after each compression to encourage venous return to the heart. In practice allowing time for recoil depends more on overall rate than technique.

Two-thumb method

- Position both thumbs over the lower third of the sternum, i.e. one finger's breadth below the inter-nipple line. The thumbs may be placed side by side or overlapping in smaller babies.
- Encircle the chest with both hands (Fig. 9.2), giving support to the baby's back.
- Apply pressure through the thumbs only. Do not put pressure on the rib cage by using a squeezing action as this makes compressions inefficient and may cause trauma.
- Perform compressions at the depth and rate prescribed above.

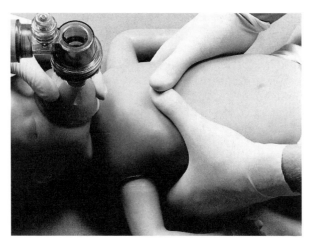

Fig. 9.2 Chest compression – two-thumb method

Two-finger method

- For this technique the baby must be on a firm, flat surface, normally the resuscitaire.
- Place the index and middle fingers on the lower third of the sternum (Fig. 9.3).
- The fingers must be perpendicular to the chest.
- Perform compressions at the depth and rate prescribed above.

A comparison of the two methods

Current international compression recommendations include both methods, but the two-thumb method is preferred as it is the most effective. There is sufficient evidence to show that higher coronary artery perfusion pressures are produced than with the two-finger method (Todres and Rogers, 1975; David, 1988). In addition, especially if maintained for more than a few minutes, it is less fatiguing for the operator.

Nevertheless, many experienced resuscitators continue to prefer the two-finger method. It is performed standing alongside the baby, while the two-thumb method requires the operator to be placed at the feet. Modern resuscitaire design does not really help with this as leaning over the baby from the bottom end may be technically difficult,

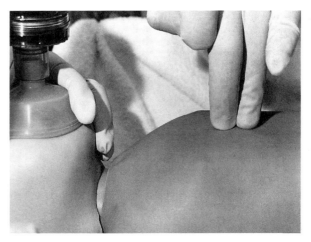

Fig. 9.3 Chest compression – two-finger method

involve uncomfortable exposure to the overhead heater and hinder access for umbilical vein catheterization. If only one experienced resuscitator is available, it is at least possible to ventilate with a tracheal tube and T-piece and perform compressions at the same time using the two-finger method.

Re-assessment of the baby

After one minute of compressions estimate the heart rate. If the rate is:

- 100 and rising, discontinue compressions and reassess respiratory activity and colour
- unchanged or falling despite adequate ventilation and chest compressions give adrenaline.

Discontinuing chest compressions

Stop chest compressions when:

- the heart rate rises to 100 or
- the resuscitation is abandoned.

Chapter summary

During newborn resuscitation a bradycardia of less than 60 beats per minute or less than 100 and falling despite adequate ventilation requires the immediate institution of cardiac compressions using either of the methods described in this chapter. After a minute of full CPR the heart rate needs to be re-evaluated and appropriate action taken.

Chapter 10

IV access and medications

Introduction

A small proportion of babies needing resuscitation fail to respond after a minute of full CPR and the heart rate remains < 60. This is an uncommon situation occurring in about 0.1% of live births (Perlman and Reiser, 1995) and is likely to be encountered only three to four times a year in the average District General Hospital with 3–4000 births. Although treatment with a number of medications and fluids may help to salvage some of these babies, the need to administer adrenaline, which is the drug of first choice, is nevertheless associated with a poor prognosis (Sims *et al.*, 1994). This is a reflection of the severity of hypoxia in babies that reach this stage.

The rationale for giving medications and fluids is to increase the cardiac output and improve cardiac and cerebral perfusion. If successful this will lead to generalized re-oxygenation and correction of the acid–base imbalance (Fig. 10.1). In addition, naloxone is of use in counteracting narcotic-induced respiratory depression and dextrose solutions may be required for hypoglycaemia.

The use of medications in the newborn is controversial and much of it based on evidence from adults. There is very little good evidence for a number of routine practices which are now enshrined in national and international guidelines.

Chapter objectives

At the end of the chapter the reader will be able to:

- list the routes available for administering medications and fluids
- outline the methods for establishing these routes

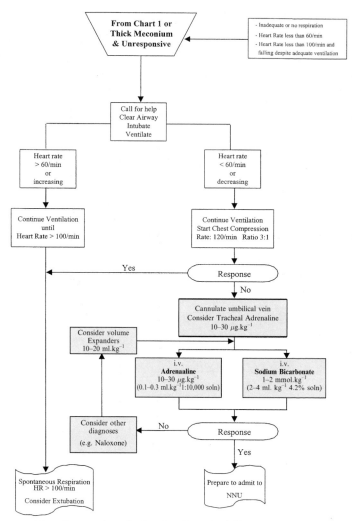

Note: Repeat adrenalin dose I.v. 100 μg.kg^{-1} if no response

Fig. 10.1 Resuscitation of the newborn chart 2

- list the medications and fluids used
- list the rationale and indications for use, preparations and doses and appropriate routes of administration for each medication and fluid.

Routes of administration

Once the decision to use medications has been made, swift administration by an appropriate route must be ensured. Advanced
resuscitators should be familiar with the following routes of access
and be adept at securing them:

- umbilical vein catheter
- tracheal tube
- intraosseous cannula
- peripheral vein cannula
- intramuscular injection.

Umbilical vein catheter

This is the preferred route for administering medication and fluids
apart from naloxone. Access can almost always be achieved very
quickly and without difficulty.

Equipment (Fig. 10.2)
Sterile gloves
Sterile gown
Sterile dressing pack
Aqueous chlorhexidine
FG4 and FG5 umbilical catheter
Three-way tap
Normal saline
10 ml syringe
Cotton tape
Artery forceps
Scalpel
Suture
Tape

Procedure
1. Think ahead. If it looks as though venous access will be required
   have the above equipment opened.
2. Wear sterile gloves and use full aseptic technique despite the
   urgency of the situation.
3. Take a FG4 or FG5 umbilical catheter, attach a three-way tap
   and flush with normal saline.

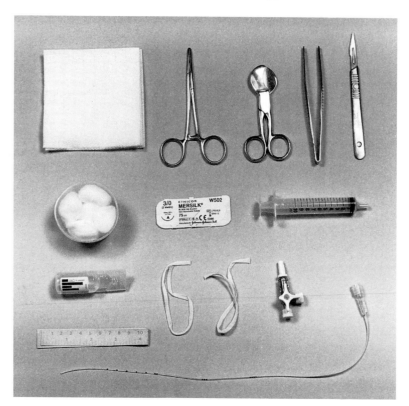

Fig. 10.2 Umbilical vein catheterization equipment

4. Grasp the cord with sterile gauze and clean it and the skin at its base with aqueous chlorhexidine.
5. Put a tape around the base of the cord to control bleeding.
6. Cut the cord approximately 2 cm from the skin.
7. Hold the cord firmly with either gauze or artery forceps. Three vessels are normally present. The single thin-walled vein can be easily identified. It may be oozing blood and is readily distinguished from the white thick-walled arteries.
8. Insert the tip of catheter into the vein 5 cm below the skin surface in a term baby. This will enable central infusion of drugs which therefore have a better chance of reaching the heart. The catheter may enter the liver or portal system and injection of drugs here may be less effective and also cause tissue damage. Without an

X-ray it may be difficult to determine if this has happened but, in general, this will result in difficulty advancing the catheter further and also in aspirating blood. This is unlikely to happen if the catheter is only inserted 5 cm.

9. Once blood flows back drugs and fluids can then be administered before it is secured. Secure with a stitch and mark with a flag as soon as is practical.

> Administration of adrenaline or naloxone directly into the umbilical cord by needle and syringe is unreliable and should be discouraged.

Tracheal tube

In an emergency situation with the baby intubated but no immediately available intravenous access, adrenaline can be given by this route. There is little evidence that this is effective in the newborn and doses 10-fold higher than the IV dose are required to achieve comparable blood levels (Lindemann, 1984).

Procedure
1. Put adrenaline dose into 5Fg feeding tube.
2. Disconnect tracheal tube.
3. Thread feeding tube down beyond the end of tracheal tube.
4. Flush adrenaline into trachea with 1 ml of normal saline.
5. Reconnect and continue ventilation.

Alternatively dilute adrenaline dose in 1–2 ml of normal saline, inject into tracheal tube, and continue ventilation.

> The tracheal route should only be used if umbilical vein access is unavailable.

Intraosseous infusion

This is a recently re-discovered method of securing rapid intravenous access in infants and children. In practice umbilical catheterization is so quick and easy that this route is rarely used. However 'if venous access fails, an intraosseous needle can be inserted into the tibia and this route used instead of the venous umbilical catheter' (European Resuscitation Council, 1998). The method for use in neonates has been described elsewhere (Ellemunter *et al.*, 1999).

Peripheral vein

This is usually the commonest site for intravenous access but in the collapsed neonate takes too long and often fails altogether.

Intracardiac injection of adrenaline is *not* recommended in any guidelines but is still practised. Unless more evidence becomes available adrenaline should be administered only by intravenous, intratracheal or possibly intraosseous routes.

Medications (Fig. 10.3)

Only a few drugs or fluids are recommended for use in neonatal resuscitation. Ideally, experienced resuscitators should be familiar with doses but, in practice, since they are infrequently used, a list of doses should be posted on the resuscitaire for the following:

- adrenaline
- 4.2% sodium bicarbonate
- volume expanders
- 10% dextrose
- naloxone hydrochloride.

Adrenaline

Adrenaline is a naturally occurring catecholamine produced by the adrenal medulla. It stimulates both alpha- and beta-receptors. Beta-receptor stimulation increases the heart rate (chronotropic effect) and force of contraction (inotropic effect). Beta$_2$ receptors stimulated at low adrenaline concentrations produce vasodilation. The main effect at the higher concentrations achieved during resuscitation is alpha stimulation which causes intense systemic vasoconstriction. The coronary and cerebral circulations are spared this effect and, as a result, their perfusion is increased (Michael *et al.*, 1984; Berkowitz *et al.*, 1989).

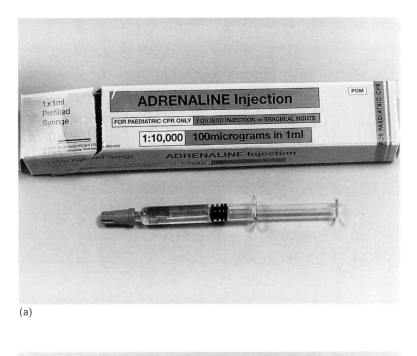

(a)

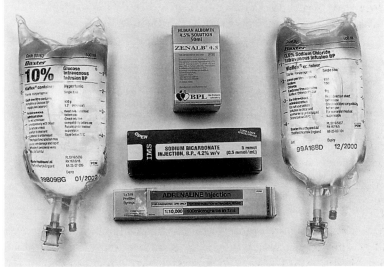

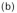
(b)

Fig. 10.3   (a) and (b) Resuscitation medication and fluids

Indications

Heart rate < 60, despite one minute of effective ventilation and chest compressions.

Preparation

1 : 10 000 solution (100 μg/ml) in 10 ml ampoule.

Dose

0.1–0.3ml/kg of 1 : 10 000 solution (10–30 μg/kg).

Some authorities (Royal College of Paediatrics and Child Health, 1997) recommend a higher dose of 100 μg/kg IV if there is no response to two boluses at the lower dose, following adult regimens. Higher dose adrenaline has not been studied in newborn resuscitation but there are some theoretical disadvantages (Pasternak *et al.*, 1983). The prognosis after no response to two lower doses of adrenaline becomes increasingly poor and the argument may turn out to be purely academic.

Route

- Umbical venous catheter
- Tracheal tube
- Intraosseous.

Sodium bicarbonate

Sodium bicarbonate is not recommended for brief periods of CPR. Once tissues are oxygenated by lung inflation with 100% oxygen and cardiac compressions, the acidosis will self-correct unless asphyxia is very severe. In prolonged arrests the development of profound acidosis depresses cardiac output and blood pressure and creates resistance to catecholamine pressor effects (Ginsburg and Goldsmith, 1998). At this point alkali may be beneficial, though there is precious little evidence for this in the newborn (Gazmuri *et al.*, 1990).

The objective of giving bicarbonate is not to correct the overall metabolic acidosis (this would take for example around 30 ml/kg at this late stage, fifteen times more than the recommended dose). If a little bicarbonate gets into the coronary arteries it might improve myocardial function. By the time adrenaline is required the prognosis is poor. Failure to respond to two doses of adrenaline means it is even worse. Not surprisingly then, few babies are likely to respond to sodium bicarbonate infusion. There is evidence from animal work that, in asphyxiated dogs, sodium bicarbonate has the paradoxical effect of causing a fall of cardiac output and blood pressure (Arieff *et al.*, 1982). In addition, concerns have been raised about the risk of intraventricular haemorrhage in preterm babies treated with intravenous sodium bicarbonate; 8.4% solutions should never be used and the bolus should be injected slowly (Finberg, 1977; Papile *et al.*, 1978; Howell, 1987). If bicarbonate is to be used these are the only practical precautions that can be taken.

Indications
Heart rate < 60 despite effective ventilation, chest compressions and two intravenous doses of adrenaline.

Preparation
4.2% solution (0.5 mmol/ml).

Dose
2–4 ml/kg (1–2 mmol/kg).

Following administration, carbon dioxide is generated and this will worsen the respiratory component of the acidosis unless it is excreted by the lungs (Ostrea and Odell, 1972). This means that full CPR must of course be maintained throughout.

Route
- Intravenous, preferably by an umbilical venous catheter.
- Intraosseous.

Volume expander

Indications
Infrequently needed in practice. Hypovolaemia leads to poor tissue perfusion and acidosis. Shock in the delivery room is usually cardiogenic secondary to hypoxia. Detecting hypovolaemia is not always easy but it should be suspected with:

- evidence of acute blood loss. This may be overt, e.g. pulmonary haemorrhage, or suspected, e.g. visceral trauma
- persistent signs of shock (pallor, tachycardia, weak peripheral pulses) despite adequate resuscitation.

NB: Anaemia due to in-utero haemolysis or fetal transfusion syndromes will usually present as severe pallor, and hyper- rather than hypovolaemia will be present. Packed cells or exchange transfusion rather than volume expanders are indicated.

Preparations
- 4.5% human albumin
- group O Rhesus negative blood. There will not be time to crossmatch blood in most situations
- 0.9% normal saline.

Despite the ongoing contoversy over the use of human albumin solution, there is currently insufficient evidence on which to base the choice between crystalloid and colloid for resuscitation. The use of human albumin solution in neonates is widespread and based on clinical experience.

Volume
- 10–20 ml/kg administered as quickly as possible in the rare event of severe hypovolaemia. This will most usually be due to fetal bleeding.
- Following administration the baby should be re-assessed. The bolus can be repeated if signs of hypovolaemia persist.
- Special care needs to be taken to avoid over-transfusion in preterm babies because they tolerate volume expansion less well and may suffer complications.

Route
- Umbilical vein catheter
- Intraosseous can also be used. This is the last situation in which you should be looking for a peripheral vein.

Dextrose

Indication
- Hypoglycaemia is not usually a problem but, if resuscitation has been prolonged, blood sugars should be measured and levels < 2.5 mmol/l treated.

There is little point in administering dextrose without checking the blood sugar first.

Preparation
10% solution.

Dose
3 ml/kg of 10% dextrose.

Route
- Umbilical vein catheter
- Intraosseous.

Naloxone hydrochloride (Narcan)

Naloxone is a narcotic antagonist that reverses the respiratory depressant effects of narcotic analgesics (mainly pethidine) used in labour. This usually occurs if pethidine has been given within a few hours prior to birth, an increasingly infrequent occurrence in modern practice. It has no respiratory depressant effect itself (Handal *et al.*, 1983).

Suspecting drug-induced respiratory depression should not distract from the first principle of resuscitation, i.e. to open the airway and ensure adequate ventilation. This is all that will usually be needed and once the baby is pink but still not breathing, naloxone should be given. The duration of action is up to 24 hours after intramuscular injection. This may be shorter than the duration of the narcotic effect and it may therefore be necessary to repeat the dose (Chernow, 1988). However, this is rarely needed in our experience.

Indications
Apnoea or inadequate respiration after the mother has been given pethidine up to 4 hours before delivery.

Preparation
Naloxone ampoule 400 μg/ml.

Dose
0.25 ml/kg of 400 μg/ml

Route
- Intramuscular injection
- Intravenous (unlikely to be available).

Naloxone should not be given to the baby of an opiate dependent mother. This is likely to precipitate acute withdrawal, often presenting with hypertonia, irritability and convulsions.

Other drugs

A number of other drugs such as calcium salts and atropine have been used in neonatal resuscitation in the past but there is a consensus that these are either of no use or actually harmful. They should not be available on the resuscitaire.

Chapter summary

Failure of asphyxiated babies to respond to full CPR indicates profound metabolic disturbance. The use of adrenaline and bicarbonate at this stage may rescue some babies, but is generally associated with a poor prognosis. Details of adrenaline and bicarbonate use have been covered. The use of volume expanders for shock, naloxone for narcotic-induced respiratory depression and dextrose for hypoglycaemia has also been outlined. Details of the various routes of administration including practical methods have been given.

Chapter 11

Special situations

Introduction

Many unusual situations may face the midwife and doctor in the delivery room. These can create diagnostic difficulties, require specific management and pose major ethical dilemmas. The resuscitation methods taught so far are an adequate basis for assessment and management, but most will need extra consideration.

Chapter objectives

At the end of this chapter the reader will be able to:

- identify nine special conditions affecting resuscitation of the newborn baby
- describe the features that are important in anticipating and recognizing these conditions
- outline the additional management required in each case.

Meconium aspiration syndrome (MAS)

Meconium-stained amniotic fluid (MSAF) is common, occurring in more than 10% of deliveries (Wiswell *et al.*, 1990). Thinly stained fluid is unlikely to cause a problem as coexisting asphyxia is unlikely. The presence of thick meconium in amniotic fluid is more likely to indicate asphyxia and hence intrapartum gasping with the possibility of meconium aspiration syndrome (MAS).

In MAS, complex processes cause areas of collapse and air trapping as a result of complete and partial small airway obstruction (Fig. 11.1). This leads to difficulty with ventilation, ventilation perfusion mismatch causing hypoxia, and may be complicated by air leaks such as pneumothorax. Chronic intrauterine hypoxia may, in addition, cause high pulmonary artery resistance resulting in persistence of the fetal circulation. In severe cases these factors may create major difficulties with resuscitation.

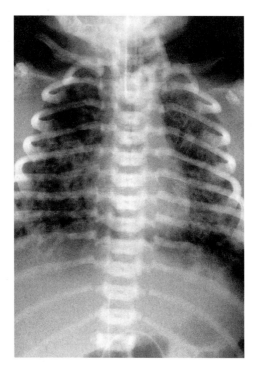

Fig. 11.1 X-ray: meconium aspiration syndrome

The following steps should be taken when thick meconium has been draining in the liquor:

- A skilled resuscitator should be present.
- As soon as the head is delivered suck out the nose and oropharynx.
- When delivery is completed remove the baby quickly to the resuscitaire.
- If the baby is vigorous, pink or rapidly improving there will

usually be no need to intubate. Suction the oropharynx. Aspiration is less likely to occur in these babies as airway protective reflexes are still present. If large quantities of meconium are aspirated it will be necessary to inspect the cords with the laryngoscope and proceed accordingly.

- If CNS depression is present, there is a strong possibility that meconium has been aspirated and intubation is required. Insert the laryngoscope and suction the pharynx under direct vision. Inspect the cords. Suction if meconium is present. Intubate. Intubation should be performed even if the cords look clear as this does not exclude aspiration. The cords were clear in the baby in Figure 11.1, but large quantities of meconium were removed from the trachea.

- Now apply suction to the tracheal tube. This can be performed in one of two ways. Suction can be applied directly through the tracheal tube. The Coles tube has a T-piece usually used for intermittent positive pressure ventilation (IPPV) which can be attached to the suction. An adapter with a side port for the straight tubes is available enabling them to be used in a similar fashion. A less satisfactory alternative is to pass the largest bore suction tube possible down the tracheal tube itself. Gently withdraw the tracheal tube or suction catheter depending on which method is being used. Very thick meconium may not pass up either tube but may be withdrawn captured on the end. After one or more withdrawals no meconium will be aspirated. At this point ventilation may be started by tube.

- Saline lavage is still practised but will not assist in the recovery of significant quantities of meconium.

- The badly asphyxiated baby with profound bradycardia poses a dilemma. Airway clearance need not be scrupulous. Oxygenation must have some priority in this situation. Quickly suction the trachea and then ventilate.

- Once ventilation has started suction the oropharynx again as meconium may well up from the stomach. Pass an NGT and empty the stomach.

- Even if particulate meconium has been aspirated from the trachea but breathing is adequate, ventilation may not be necessary. The vigorous baby with a clear airway and no respiratory distress should join his mother. Ventilated babies and those with respiratory signs should be transferred to the neonatal unit as soon as they are stable.

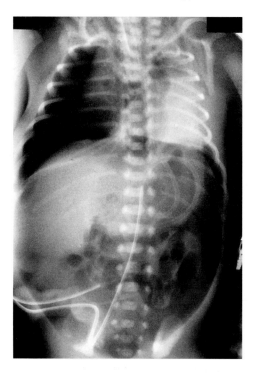

Fig. 11.2 Tension pneumothorax (this should normally be diagnosed before the X-ray is taken!)

Pneumothorax

Incidence

Simple pneumothorax is relatively common, but is usually asymptomatic and often goes undetected. Fortunately tension pneumothorax (Fig. 11.2) is rare during resuscitation, but when it does occur it is a potentially life-threatening condition requiring rapid diagnosis and treatment.

It may occur with:

- MAS
- diaphragmatic hernia
- over-enthusiastic positive pressure ventilation
- no apparent reason.

Presenting signs

Tension pneumothorax presents as an initial difficulty with resuscitation or a subsequent deterioration which may cause acute cardio-respiratory collapse. The main clinical signs vary with severity and include:

- Over-inflated chest with little or no movement especially on the side of pneumothorax.
- Absent breath sounds on the side of lesion, and in extreme cases on both sides or bilateral pneumothorax.
- Apex beat displaced to unaffected side.
- Increased resistance to ventilation.
- Abdominal distension.

Management

With acute collapse suspected to be due to pneumothorax, cold light examination can be performed if immediately available. Otherwise insert a 21G(green) butterfly attached to a three-way tap and 10 ml syringe into the third intercostal space in the midclavicular line. If a pneumothorax is present air will be aspirated easily. Air will not be aspirated from a normal lung. The risk of actually causing a tension pneumothorax by 'needling' the chest is very small, but this should not encourage its indiscriminate use.

Relief of the pneumothorax will enable the resuscitation to proceed. Occasional repeated aspirations may be required until a chest drain can be inserted.

Diaphragmatic hernia

In this condition abdominal contents, especially stomach and gut, herniate through the diaphragm into the chest (Fig. 11.3). This occurs in early gestation and causes at least some degree of lung hypoplasia.

Incidence

Incidence is about 1:4000 live births. In 80% of cases the defect is left sided. Many cases are now diagnosed by antenatal ultrasound, but unanticipated cases are still encountered in the delivery room. The mortality is still high in either case at around 50% (Langham *et al.*, 1996).

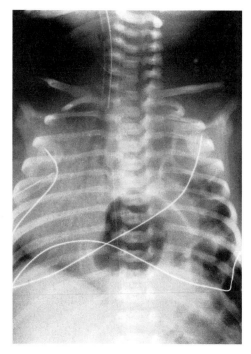

Fig. 11.3 X-ray: diaphragmatic hernia

Presenting signs

The usual clinical signs are:

- respiratory distress with cyanosis (Fig. 11.4)
- scaphoid (concave) abdomen
- heart deviated to the right (left-sided cases)
- absent breath sounds on affected side.

Occasional asymptomatic cases are detected by X-ray.

In cases diagnosed antenatally, delivery should be planned at a regional unit closely linked to the paediatric surgical unit.

Resuscitation

- Intubate and ventilate. This will usually but not always be immediately necessary. Under no circumstances ventilate by face mask if the diagnosis is even suspected. This will inflate stomach

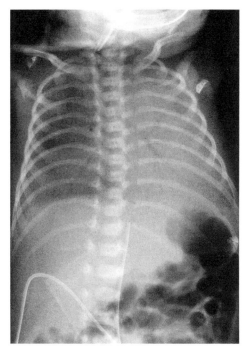

Fig. 11.4 X-ray: respiratory distress syndrome
(note the tracheal tube is about to fall out)

and bowel, increasing respiratory embarrassment. Higher ventilation pressures will then be required. This increases the risk of pneumothorax.

- Pass a large (10 or 12 FG) nasogastric tube and leave on free drainage.
- Paralysis and analgesia may be required before transfer to the neonatal unit. Other details such as immediate ventilator management and treating pulmonary hypertension are beyond the scope of this chapter.

Hydrops fetalis

Incidence

The commonest cause of this was once Rhesus disease with antenatal haemolytic anaemia causing cardiac failure. Since the introduction of anti-D immunoglobulin and antenatal detection and management of affected fetuses, this is rare. Non-isoimmune cases occur due to a variety of causes, most commonly cardiac disease and chromosomal abnormalities. Some of these are detected antenatally by ultrasound but some still present as an unpleasant surprise at delivery. The overall incidence is about 1:3000 live births. There is a high mortality in severely affected babies and resuscitation will be difficult.

Clinical presentation

This condition is easily recognized. The main features are pallor, generalized oedema, ascites and pleural effusions.

Resuscitation

- If the diagnosis is recognized antenatally ensure there are two resuscitators present.
- Put the baby on the resuscitaire in a foot-down position to minimize the mechanical effect of the ascites on breathing. This position is difficult to achieve on most resuscitaires. Intubation and ventilation using high pressures will be required immediately.
- Tense ascites will require draining if ventilation is difficult. Site a cannula in the left iliac fossa. This will prevent damage to the liver and spleen, which are usually enlarged.
- Drain fluid slowly until ventilation becomes easier. The cannula can then be removed. In practice pleural effusions do not usually limit ventilation but, if they do, drain as for a pneumothorax.
- Severe anaemia and/or hypervolaemia are likely to be present. Insert umbilical vein catheter. Send blood for urgent haematocrit, etc. A packed cell transfusion of 10–20 ml of O negative blood can be given but an exchange transfusion with whole blood is more likely to be effective.
- In the most desperate circumstances this may need to be done in the delivery room. Remove 20 ml of blood. Replace with 10 ml of O negative whole blood. Do a single volume (85 ml/kg) exchange transfusion and leave the 10 ml deficit standing at the end. Ideally this will be done in intensive care.

Acute blood loss

Incidence

Significant fetal blood loss is uncommon now with the virtual disappearance of obstetric trauma. It does still occur, however, as a result of haemorrhage from the fetal side of the placenta, cord and in acute forms of feto–maternal and twin–twin transfusion syndromes.

Clinical presentation

Babies have a circulating blood volume of about 85 ml/kg. A 20% loss of circulating volume (a mere 50 ml in a term baby) will produce signs of shock:

- tachycardia
- low volume pulses
- poor capillary refill
- pallor
- poor response to resuscitation.

Resuscitation

The management is airway and breathing, then circulation as usual. Once adequate ventilation is established catheterize the umbilical vein and infuse 20 ml/kg of O negative blood. This can be syringed in quickly in a badly shocked baby but more slowly, over 10 minutes, in less severe cases. Reassess the circulation after completion. The volume may need to be repeated but this would imply an initial loss of 50% circulating volume or ongoing loss.

Upper airway obstruction

A number of rare cases of upper airway obstruction present as resuscitation emergencies at birth. *Choanal atresia,* in which the nasal passages are obstructed by either a bony or a cartilaginous septum, is the commonest. Since the neonate is an obligate nose breather this may produce failure to breathe at birth. Recovery will be rapid with crying, face mask ventilation or after intubation, but apnoea recurs during quiet independent breathing. The diagnosis should be confirmed by failure to pass a suction catheter through the nose. About half of these babies have choanal atresia as one of a number of abnormalities making up the CHARGE syndrome:

*C*olobomata of the eyes
*H*eart disease
*A*tresia of the choanae

*R*etarded growth and development
*G*enital hypoplasia (males)
*E*ar deformities.

An oral airway may enable normal breathing, otherwise intubation will be required until an ENT opinion has been obtained.

Tumours and congenital malformations of the upper airway, such as Pierre–Robin syndrome, may also cause life-threatening obstructions at birth. These may be very difficult to deal with and again require the help of an experienced ENT surgeon.

Fetal abnormality

Many serious fetal abnormalities are detected antenatally by AFP and ultrasound screening. This is likely to increase in future and enables the delivery and management to be planned with parental involvement. In those cases where termination is not an issue or the parents decide against it, a named midwife should be involved in these discussions and ideally be present at delivery to provide continuity of support. The paediatrician who has been involved earlier should be present at the delivery or at least be aware that it is taking place. The newborn with severe undiagnosed abnormalities presents special problems.

- Babies with anencephaly and other lethal abnormalities will need no resuscitation but pose a major challenge in our ability to assist sensitively in a human tragedy.
- In general, other babies should be resuscitated and transferred to the neonatal unit for further care and diagnostic investigations. There may be little or no relationship between cosmetic appearance and the long-term prognosis.
- Abnormal babies who are difficult to resuscitate need the most senior paediatrician available to advise on diagnosis, prognosis and management.

Extreme prematurity

24–28 weeks' gestation

The general principles of resuscitation are no different to those already outlined. The following points need to be noted however:

- Special care needs to be taken to prevent heat loss. Low admission temperature in this group of babies is directly related to survival.
- Many of these babies will require respiratory support because of premature lung disease, especially if no dexamethasone has been given to the mother. Therefore support ventilation more readily if breathing looks inadequate. Specific suggestions include face mask ventilation for failure to cry by 15 seconds or to breathe by 30 seconds and intubation if not breathing after a further 30 seconds (European Resuscitation Council, 1998).
- Intubation will often be needed without delay. This will enable better control over pressure (start with 30 cm H_2O) and also allow longer inspiratory times which are required for the first few breaths. Those babies will also require the first dose of surfactant down the tracheal tube. This can be given as soon as the lungs are inflated.
- Subsequent ventilation pressures should be the minimum to produce good chest movement and oxygenation. At the present there is no way of giving positive end expiratory pressure (PEEP) in the delivery room to help prevent the lungs collapsing at the end of expiration. This is especially likely if surfactant has not been given.
- Transfer directly to the neonatal unit ensuring that the baby is not allowed to get cold or hypoxic en route.

Less than 24 weeks' gestation

This is a very difficult group technically, ethically and legally. They are technically below the level of viability but are quite often born alive. Also, while the mortality is very high, as is the handicap rate in survivors, a few do survive relatively intact. One year results of the EPICURE study of babies born before 26 weeks' gestation show only 11% of survivors apparently normal at the first birthday.

Local written guidelines are recommended for this group of babies. These are often of necessity rather vague but should cover the following:

- Babies at this interface of survival (and their parents) should be given the benefit of receiving the services of the paediatricians.
- Such cases should be discussed with the senior paediatrician on-call. Depending on whether the delivery is anticipated or

completed, the paediatrician may visit the parents beforehand or give advice on or come to see the baby.

- Badly bruised babies and those who do not respond quickly to resuscitation, especially if they require compressions or adrenaline, have effectively no chance of survival.

Some paediatricians will consider only those babies who are vigorous at least initially or responsive to minimal resuscitation such as face mask ventilation as suitable for further medical care.

Inasmuch as is possible all parties including parents and members of the medical and midwifery team should agree that the best course of action has been taken. This is usually not difficult to achieve in practice.

Multiple births

Twins and higher order births present special problems in resuscitation at birth. In modern obstetric practice twins and triplets are almost always diagnosed. This gives ample opportunity to plan the delivery especially with the resuscitation in mind. Undiagnosed twins may pose special problems (Bryan, 1992).

Multiple births should all take place in an obstetric unit with a capacity for at least short-term neonatal intensive care. This requires one set of equipment, including resuscitaires, for each baby. One paediatrician with advanced life support skills also needs to be immediately available for each baby. This is especially important out of normal working hours. An intensive care cot should be available for each baby. Apart from the obvious numerical problem a number of perinatal complications are much commoner in multiple than single births:

- Prematurity. Generally the more fetuses present the earlier labour is likely to commence.
- Malpresentation. Less than 50% of twins present by the vertex. About a third present by the breech. Other malpresentations are common. The caesarean section rate is high. In addition, the less common problem of fetal locking may occur.
- Transfusion syndrome. Twin–twin transfusion syndrome (Fig. 11.5) may occur chronically or more acutely during the delivery resulting in one overtransfused and one anaemic or hypovolaemic

twin each of which may prove difficult to resuscitate.
- The second twin. The mortality in the second twin may reach up to ten times that of the overall perinatal mortality. Hypoxia is largely responsible for this.

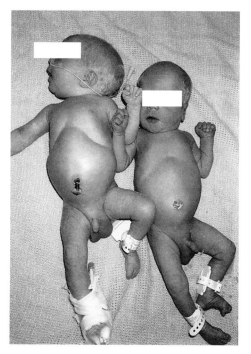

Fig. 11.5 Twin transfusion syndrome

Chapter summary

Nine special situations which can create diagnostic difficulties, require specific management and pose major ethical dilemmas have been discussed in respect of resuscitation. Extra consideration regarding resuscitation methods and interventions have been outlined.

Chapter 12

Post-resuscitation care and transport

Introduction

Babies who have received minimal resuscitation can normally be handed straight to their mothers. Little extra post-resuscitation care may be necessary and may consist of no more than attention to keeping the baby warm, initiation of feeding and some routine observations of colour, respiration and temperature. This can be provided on the postnatal ward.

However, babies who have required more extensive and prolonged resuscitation will need more care, close observation and often electrical monitoring. Such babies are usually admitted to the neonatal unit (Fig. 12.1). This may require transfer only a short distance away in the same hospital or sometimes some miles by road to a regional neonatal unit. The purpose of this chapter is to provide an outline of the principles of safe and effective post-resuscitation care and transport for these babies who require more advanced care on a neonatal unit.

Chapter objectives

At the end of this chapter the reader will be able to:

- list the main priorities of stabilization
- list the resuscitation-related criteria for admission to a neonatal unit
- outline necessary communications with the receiving unit and with the parents
- list equipment used in transport over a distance
- list the problems associated with transit
- describe the care given in transit and the handover given to the receiving unit.

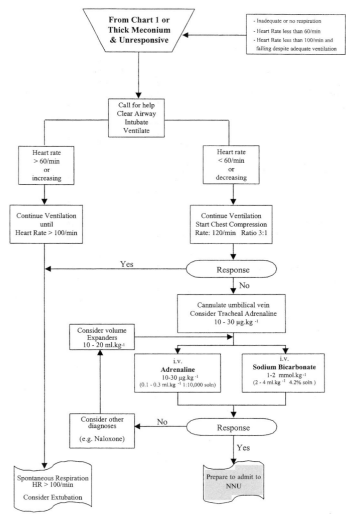

Note: Repeat adrenalin dose I.v. $100\,\mu g.kg^{-1}$ if no response

Fig. 12.1 Resuscitation of the newborn chart 2

Priorities of stabilization

Keeping the baby stable in the immediate post-resuscitation period is as important as the resuscitation itself. In addition, rapid detection of any deterioration in the clinical condition is essential. Routine general observation and monitoring of the heart and respiratory rates and temperature should continue at intervals determined by the clinical condition. Pulse oximetry providing continuous information on heart rate and oxygen saturations in a non-invasive way is useful and can be commenced in the delivery suite. In this way deterioration can be anticipated or detected early and appropriate action taken. Maintaining normal temperature, a clear airway, adequate ventilation and normal circulation are the initial priorities. Once these are controlled other matters that may need attention include:

- definitive securing of tracheal tube
- X-ray to check tube position
- establishment of venous access if not already achieved
- laboratory investigations, e.g. blood glucose, blood culture, electrolytes, clotting studies, etc.
- treatment of hypoglycaemia if detected on BM testing
- any other specific treatments indicated, e.g. antibiotics
- vitamin K 1 mg IM in line with local policy.

Criteria for admission to the neonatal unit

All neonatal units should have their own policies covering admission criteria. Some of these refer to neonatal conditions not related to resuscitation, e.g. infants of diabetic mothers, prematurity and intrauterine growth retardation, but a number relate specifically to resuscitation:

- prolonged resuscitation
- continuing need for additional oxygen or respiratory support
- meconium aspiration
- some congenital abnormalities, e.g. diaphragmatic hernia.

It must be stressed that only babies that need extra care should be transferred to the neonatal unit. This is an obvious but, nevertheless, necessary point. Any such admission carries the following consequences:

- Emotionally painful separation from the mother. Although this may not result in the serious problems with mother–infant bonding that were once suspected (Klaus and Kennel, 1976) it is still an important consideration.

- Disempowerment of the parents as their roles are taken over by neonatal staff. This may delay the development of the parents' confidence in becoming the primary carers (Yeo, 1998).
- High cost of neonatal cots. These are often also in short supply.
- Risk of transfer itself, especially to a distant site.
- Increased risk of nosocomial infection.

Transfer within the hospital

The following general principles should be adhered to:

- Label the baby.
- Do not transfer until the baby is fully stabilized.
- Make sure that tracheal tubes, intravenous lines, etc. are properly secured.
- Check that the neonatal unit is fully prepared to receive the baby.
- Transfer the baby in a transport incubator or on the resuscitaire depending on the local situation.
- Ensure that the baby does not become cold or hypoxic during transfer. Remember the resuscitaire overhead heater will not be working once unplugged, therefore make sure the baby is adequately covered.
- Do not delay transfer unnecessarily.
- Keep the parents fully informed.

Transfer to another hospital

Arrangements for transport will vary. In some areas organized retrieval teams from regional centres will be responsible for transfer, while in others it will fall to the referring hospital. This may be especially the case if the transfer is necessary because of cardiac or surgical problems.

Problems of transfer

The aim must be to provide the same standard of care during transfer as would be given in the neonatal unit. The difficulties in ensuring this are due to:

- The environment. There is as yet no ideal transfer vehicle or transport incubator. Space is limited in the vehicles used and also in the transport incubators which are smaller than standard incubators. Problems occur particularly in winter with lower ambient temperature, and both noise and movement may cause extra difficulties. These factors may interfere with both clinical and electronic monitoring of the baby. It will also make any procedures such as reintubation, etc. more difficult.
- The equipment. This is often different to that in routine use. There are potential problems with oxygen, air and power supplies. Equipment that fails during transfer may be difficult to replace.
- The team. The restriction on space usually means that only one doctor and one nurse/midwife will be present. The back up available in hospital is temporarily unavailable.
- The baby. Premature and sick babies, i.e. the ones most likely to be transferred, are particularly vulnerable to the hazards of transfer (Leslie and Stephenson, 1998).
- The parents. Parents will have to travel separately from their baby and it may sometimes be impossible for the mother to be transferred to the same hospital, at least immediately.

Transfer with the currently available technology is obviously far from ideal and everything must be done to prevent it being needed. This includes the concentration of births of high-risk neonates in centres with neonatal intensive care facilities and especially in-utero transfer of babies less than 28 weeks' gestation.

Communication with the receiving unit

The following information needs to be provided:

- Baby details. Name, date and time of birth, gestation, weight, diagnoses, resuscitation details.
- Respiratory status. Diagnoses, respiratory rate, recession, etc., FiO_2, ventilator settings.
- Haemodynamic status. Heart rate, blood pressures, fluid therapy, inotropes, etc.
- Metabolic status. Blood glucose, acid–base, etc.
- Other investigations. Blood cultures sent, etc.

- Other treatment. Antibiotics, etc.
- Parental details. Include any relevant details. Send maternal blood for crossmatching and consent for operation if appropriate. Also a brief account of what the parents have been told and whether or not they will be accompanying the baby is important.

Communication with parents

The parents will need a full but uncluttered account of the baby's problems and management. While care must be taken to avoid unnecessarily alarming the parents, a frank account of the baby's condition must be given. If transfer, especially to another hospital, is necessary they will need an explanation as to why. It is all too easy for medical and midwifery staff familiar with such transfers to assume that the need for transfer is self-evident. The parents must be allowed to play as full and informed a part as possible in the decision making at this stage. However, in practice, parents look to the professionals for advice on this matter.

Equipment required for transfer

Transport incubator (Fig. 12.2)

Several commercial incubators are available. These should include a number of essential features:

- comfortable, secure environment
- adequate room even for larger babies
- internal power supply with charge indicator and be able to use an external power supply
- an internal air/oxygen supply
- a neonatal ventilator
- monitors for heart rate, respiratory rate, oximetry and continuous monitoring of the incubator temperature and baby temperature
- small enough and sufficiently mobile to be manoeuvred by two people.

Other equipment including infusion pumps and a self-inflating bag for hand ventilation will be required. Booth (1996) gives a long list of

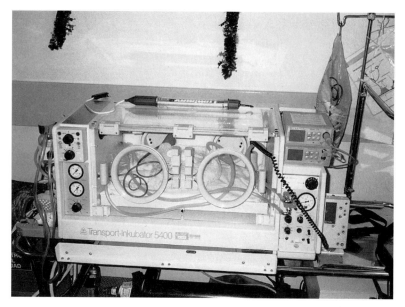

Fig. 12.2 Transport incubator

recommended ancillary equipment and drugs. Some of these may be superfluous but it is better to be over rather than under prepared.

Airway

Oxygen and air supply, hoses and connectors
Face masks (various sizes)
Oral airways (000, 00, 0, 1, 2)
Self-inflating rebreathing bag with pressure limiting valve and/or occluding T-piece with blow-off valve
Tracheal tubes (2.0, 2.5, 3.0, 3.5, 4.0, 4.5) with introducers
8 mm and 15 mm connectors and adaptors
Laryngoscopes
Magill forceps
Nasogastric tube
Suction device and catheters
Blade or scissors to cut tube to size
Tape and harness to secure tracheal tube.

Vascular access

IV cannulae – various
Butterflies and needles – various
Stylets
T-pieces
Connectors and tubing
Syringes – various
Three-way taps
Capillary tubes
Blood bottles and BM stix
Tape and splints to secure cannulae
(Intraosseous needles)
(Central catheters – UAC 3.5F, 5F and UVC 6F, 8F).

Procedures

Gloves
Scalpels
Alcohol wipes, swabs, cotton wool
Sterile saline for flushes
Cutdown set
Chest drain set with Heimlich valves
UAC, UVC set
Lumbar puncture needles
Sutures (if not in sets)
Tape, etc.

Drugs

Adrenaline
Sodium bicarbonate
Atropine
Prostin E2
Dobutamine
Plasma
Dextrose
Phenobarbitone/phenytoin
Pancuronium
Morphine
Antibiotics
Dopamine

Miscellaneous

Torch
Spare batteries for laryngoscopes etc.
Maps
Paperwork – information for parents, ward documentation
Mobile phone

Chapter summary

Babies who have needed resuscitation and who require admission to the neonatal unit need to be stabilized before being moved. The principles of stabilization have been outlined. Once this has been achieved the baby must be transferred in a safe way which avoids, as much as possible, any deterioration in the condition. Details of transfer within the hospital and to distant sites have been given. Parental involvement has been stressed.

Chapter 13

Resuscitation at home

A woman giving birth at home or in a midwife/GP unit away from the general hospital should feel confident that the midwife and doctor, if present, is able to provide help efficiently and effectively in an acute emergency prior to the transfer of the mother and baby to the general hospital (Department of Health, 1993)

Introduction

In the 1960s approximately 25% of all deliveries were home births. However, following the centralization of maternity services within hospitals, this situation has now changed. Home deliveries now amount to less than 2% of the total number of births (Office for National Statistics, 1994).

If problems do arise, it is of course important to resuscitate the baby effectively and ensure that if required, a rapid, safe transfer to hospital is arranged. Although resuscitation of a newborn baby outside the hospital environment follows the same principles and guidelines described throughout this book, there are certain considerations and potential difficulties which need to be emphasized. The aim of this chapter is to discuss these and make suggestions to help minimize the risk and optimize the success of resuscitation at home.

Chapter objectives

At the end of this chapter the reader will be able to:

- identify the potential difficulties with resuscitating a baby at home
- discuss the important aspects of preparation including risk management, good communication with the parents and provision of resuscitation equipment

- describe the resuscitation procedure with particular reference to adaptations for the home environment
- discuss the importance of transfer arrangements and the back-up services
- discuss the training needs for professionals responsible for home deliveries.

Potential difficulties associated with resuscitation at home

There are a number of potential difficulties with resuscitating a baby at home:

- limited facilities and equipment
- lack of immediately available assistance, particularly now that obstetric and paediatric flying squads are rarely available
- practitioners attending home births may have limited experience in resuscitation
- transfer to hospital may be delayed.

It is important to minimize these difficulties by ensuring adequate preparation, effective resuscitation procedure, rapid and safe transfer to hospital if required and regular staff training. These will now be discussed in turn.

Preparation

Adequate preparation is essential for all home births. It involves ensuring that:

- wherever possible high-risk deliveries take place in hospital
- good communication between the mother and the midwife is established and maintained
- the necessary resuscitation equipment is available.

Risk management

It is important to ensure that, whenever possible, for planned home deliveries there are no breaches of low obstetric risk criteria. Therefore 'local evidence-based protocols defining low obstetric risk criteria need to be developed by hospital and community staff, and user groups should also be involved in the process' (Confidential Enquiry into Stillbirths and Deaths in Infancy, 1998). Where sound selection procedures for home deliveries are in place:

- the subsequent risk for term babies is minimal, with no more than 0.2% needing more than basic resuscitation (British Paediatric Association, 1993)
- a practitioner present at the birth who has received the necessary training and gained experience in resuscitation techniques could be expected to provide appropriate resuscitation in 99% of term deliveries for which it is necessary (Department of Health, 1993).

However not all home deliveries will be in the low obstetric risk category:

- All women are entitled to an informed choice and should have access to written evidence-based literature, e.g. the MIDIRS Informed Choice leaflet. Some women in the high-risk categories may choose to deliver at home, contrary to medical and midwifery advice.
- High obstetric risk deliveries, that are being planned to be undertaken in hospital, may occur unexpectedly at home. Two recent studies suggest that 15–35% of home deliveries are unplanned (North West Thames Annual Maternity Figures, 1992, 1993; Davies *et al.*, 1996).

Good midwife–mother communication

If resuscitation is to be successful, the midwife needs to be present at the delivery. Good communication between her and the mother is therefore essential. This will also help to gain the mother's confidence. When reviewing home births which were associated with either stillbirths or neonatal deaths, the Confidential Enquiry into Stillbirths and Deaths in Infancy (1998) identified the following communication problems:

- mother had difficulty contacting the midwife once labour had started
- hospital-based midwife was unfamiliar with the remote location of the mother's home
- mother waited 5 hours before contacting the midwife
- prolonged rupture of membranes – the midwife was not informed.

To ensure good communication between the mother and the midwife the following is recommended:

- The mother should have access to a telephone in the house. If there is no terrestrial phone it would be well worth considering hiring a mobile phone, though the possibility of a poor reception should be considered.
- The midwife should ensure that the mother knows how and also when it is necessary to call her.
- Midwives attending home births should have their own mobile phone or pager.
- A 'reserve' midwife should be easily reached if the named one is not immediately available – again the mother should know how to contact her.
- A 'dry run' may be particularly helpful for planned deliveries in remote areas to ensure that the midwife is familiar with directions (this would also benefit the emergency services).

Resuscitation equipment

Appropriate equipment for resuscitation should be available and regularly checked and maintained following manufacturers' recommendations. This is particularly important for home deliveries because finding replacement parts or missing items is more difficult than in hospital. The following is a suggested list for resuscitation equipment needed for home deliveries (Royal College of Paediatrics and Child Health, 1997):

- access to a mobile home or telephone within the home
- a room heater and good light
- an appropriate padded surface at table height
- towels and gloves
- self-inflating resuscitation bag, valve and face masks 0, 00 and 000
- suction device and catheters
- resuscitation flow chart
- stop watch
- stethoscope
- oxygen cylinder with regulated flow rate of up to 10 l/min and an adjustable pressure release valve within the system
- syringes, needles and disposal box
- checklist
- torch.

A resuscitation bag, complete with equipment inventory, is ideal e.g. the 'Exmouth Bag'.

Resuscitation procedure in the home

The procedure for resuscitation at home follows the ERC guidelines discussed in this book. In particular the following should be noted:

Personnel

It is recommended that no home delivery takes place without two trained professionals present (e.g. midwife and GP or two midwives), one of whom must be proficient at face mask resuscitation (Department of Health, 1993). In practice, however, occasionally only one professional may be present, which is less than ideal.

Environment

As with in-hospital deliveries measures should be taken to minimize heat loss. These should include closing all windows and using a heater in the room. In addition, warm dry towels should be available to dry the baby. Lighting has a habit of fading at the most inconvenient times – always have a good torch at hand!

Equipment

The resuscitation equipment should be laid out in an organized fashion and ready to use (Fig. 13.1). A table of a suitable height can be used as a resuscitation surface. The possible need for resuscitation should be explained to the mother before delivery.

Early detection of problems

The fetal heart rate should be carefully monitored. A fetal Doppler should be available to determine the presence of a heart rate if it is difficult to locate or if fetal distress is suspected.

Transfer arrangements

Difficulties with transfer

The 1998 Confidential Enquiry into Stillbirths and Deaths in Infancy Report identified problems with transfer including:

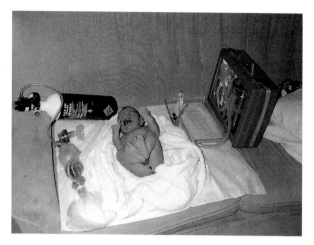

Fig. 13.1

- mother and baby sent to A & E rather than the Delivery Suite
- delayed transfer due to waiting for arrival of GP to make decision
- poor communication with the delivery suite.

Delays in transfer can affect the prognosis. It is important to ensure that when indicated, transfer of the baby to hospital is undertaken rapidly and safely.

Guidelines for transfer

It is essential that 'clear guidelines are drawn up and agreed for neonatal emergencies occurring in the community. These should cover immediate care and transfer to the neonatal unit (Department of Health, 1993).

As soon as it is indicated, arrangements should be made for transfer by whichever practitioner is present. If the midwife feels that transfer is necessary and the mother agrees, then it should be undertaken as quickly as possible and normally time should not be wasted waiting for the GP to arrive and confirm the decision.

Emergency services

The emergency services should be informed of all home births and if the house is in an isolated location a 'dry run' is advisable. The Department of Health (1993) recommend that:

- 'back-up services in the community need to be of the highest possible standard which is practical. It is essential that a comprehensive review of the system for dealing with emergencies is undertaken in every health district and local policies put into place
- each district's emergency ambulance crews should...be ready to provide such assistance as necessary to the midwife during the woman's transfer to hospital when a complication has occurred.'

Transfer priorities

When transferring the baby to hospital, the priorities should include monitoring and supporting as necessary the airway, breathing and circulation. In addition, great care should be taken to ensure the baby is kept warm. The required resuscitation equipment should also be at hand.

Training

The need to resuscitate at a home delivery is very rare and consequently practitioners in attendance may have limited resuscitation experience. Therefore, it is most important that training in newborn resuscitation is undertaken on a regular basis (see Chapter 17). At least one of the practitioners present must be competent at face mask resuscitation (British Paediatric Association, 1993).

Chapter summary

An increasing number of women are now opting for home births. The potential difficulties associated with home births have been discussed together with measures that should be taken to help minimize the risk of problems. In addition, the resuscitation procedure in the home environment has been discussed and the principles of safe transfer highlighted.

Chapter 14

Records and record keeping

Introduction

An accurate written record detailing the resuscitation events is essential, not only because it forms an integral part of the medical and midwifery management of the baby, but also because it can help to protect the practitioners if defence of their actions is required.

Unfortunately, the exact timing and sequence of events and interventions, which are particularly pertinent in newborn resuscitation, can sometimes be difficult to recall. Nevertheless, despite this, accurate record keeping will still be expected. The purpose of this chapter is to discuss some of the principles of good record keeping with particular reference to newborn resuscitation.

Chapter objectives

At the end of the chapter the reader will be able to:

- discuss the importance of accurate record keeping
- outline the principles of effective record keeping
- detail what post-resuscitation records should include
- discuss why Apgar scores should not be used as a substitute for full documentation
- discuss when the records become a legal document.

Importance of accurate record keeping

Accurate record keeping will help to protect the welfare of both the patient and practitioner by promoting:

- high standards of clinical care

- continuity of care through better communication and dissemination of information between members of the inter-professional health care team
- the ability to detect problems, such as changes in the patient's or client's condition at an early stage
- an accurate written account of treatment enabling planning and delivery of further care.

Principles of effective record keeping

According to the UKCC (1998a) there are a number of factors which contribute to effective record keeping.

The records should:

- be factual, consistent and accurate
- be documented as soon as possible after the event, providing current information on the care and condition of the baby
- be documented clearly and in such a way that the text cannot be erased
- have any alterations and additions dated, timed and signed with all original entries clearly legible
- be accurately dated, timed and signed (including a printed signature)
- not include abbreviations, jargon, meaningless phrases, irrelevant speculation.

Resuscitation records – what to include

It is most important that the resuscitation attempt is fully documented in the notes. It is recommended (Royal College of Paediatrics and Child Health, 1997) that these records should include:

- times to first gasp, regular respirations and heart rate
- details of resuscitation including response
- tracheal intubation time and duration of ventilation
- details of drugs administered, including doses and route
- umbilical cord pH, blood gases and base deficit results
- names of personnel, including designation, present

- reasons for any delay in resuscitation
- details of communication with the parents.

Clinical records should be legible and accurately reflect what happened during the resuscitation attempt. A standardized form for recording resuscitation events may help ensure that a complete record is made.

The Apgar score and documentation

The Royal College of Paediatrics and Child Health and the Royal College of Obstetricians and Gynaecologists (1997) strongly recommend that:

- the Apgar score (see Table 5.1) is not a substitute for fully documented records
- the individual observations in the Apgar scores should be recorded in full and documented at the time.

Babies with the same Apgar score may have very different problems requiring different management.

Records as a legal document

There is often concern as to what constitutes a legal document. Any document requested by the court becomes a legal document (Dimond, 1994), e.g. midwifery records, medical records, X-rays, laboratory reports, in fact any document which may be relevant to the case. If any of the documents are missing, the writer of the records may be cross-examined as to the circumstances of their disappearance (Dimond, 1994).

> medical records are not proof of the truth of the facts stated in them but the maker of the records may be called to give evidence as to the truth as to what is contained in them (Dimond, 1994)

Chapter summary

The importance of accurate records following a resuscitation attempt cannot be stressed enough. The records must be:

- factual
- legible
- clear
- concise
- accurate
- signed, timed and dated.

Chapter 15

Bereavement at birth

... and many will rejoice at his birth.
(Luke's Gospel chapter 1, verse 14.)

Introduction

Most births approach, rightly, with an expectation of joy. There is a distressing poignancy therefore when birth and death coincide. The major determinants of grief are well described in standard texts (Murray Parkes, 1986). Many of these cannot be helped or influenced in the acute situation, but everything that can be done to minimize the trauma of the event and provide effective support to the parents must be done.

The purpose of this short chapter is not to give a detailed account of neonatal bereavement, this can be found in existing works (Stewart and Dent, 1994). Rather the aim is to highlight some important practical points relating to the parental bereavement occasioned by either unsuccessful resuscitation or deliberate non-resuscitation.

Antecedent events

Sudden unexpected death, all other things being equal, is a more painful experience than anticipated death. Therefore in situations (e.g. extreme prematurity) where death soon after birth is likely, the paediatrician should, where possible, visit parents and discuss the delivery with them. This will normally be requested by the obstetricians depending on the gestation of the pregnancy. Expectations for survival are sometimes unrealistically high in very premature babies and it is often best for a paediatrician to be involved if a live birth is anticipated.

This is an important meeting and both parents and the mother's named midwife should be present. The meeting should be conducted in as unhurried a fashion as possible and should be fully documented. The location must be quiet and private. The parents need:

- accurate information about prognosis
- to be actively engaged in any decisions or plans made
- a brief account about what to expect at the delivery. 'We will be taking your baby straight to the resuscitaire for assessment and treatment if that is indicated. This will take place in the same room as your delivery. We will be busy with the baby at first but as soon as possible we will be telling you what the situation is'
- to know what their baby may be like at birth and that there may be some initial gasping. They need to be reassured that if there are signs of life initially the baby's subsequent dying will not be a violent or frightening process
- to discuss the holding of their baby at birth. Where there is hesitation over this, its importance needs to be emphasized but parents should not be pressurized
- to be reassured that the baby will not be suffering
- to be given adequate opportunity to ask questions and express fears, which may be quite different to the professional's expectations.

Despite the distressing situation most parents subsequently express gratitude for this explanation.

It is important that, where it is agreed that resuscitation will almost certainly not be appropriate, that parents are not left feeling that they have the sole responsibility for that decision. This will inevitably complicate any subsequent bereavement. The parents are now in a position to make some mental preparation for possible loss. They will now experience a degree of control in a situation that would otherwise be completely out of control for them. They will have greater confidence in the medical and nursing team despite the likely adverse outcome.

Mode of death

In most units the resuscitation will take place in the same room as the delivery. Depending on the mother's condition (anaesthesia, analgesia, natural childbirth), she will be more or less aware that the resuscitation is going on. The father, if present, may be to some extent distracted by the mother's condition, but will be similarly aware. This situation demands calm and competence. There is no need for hushed voices as long as phrases such as 'there's no heartbeat' are avoided. Neither volume nor intonation should betray anxiety. To express irritation at either one of the team or the equipment is unwise to say the least.

Breaking bad news

If, after assessment, a decision is made not to resuscitate or if resuscitation is ineffective and therefore discontinued, it is now necessary to tell the parents. In most cases they will have realized what is happening before they are told. The fact of the baby's death must be communicated in the most unambiguous but sympathetic manner possible. A simple expression such as 'I'm sorry, your baby has died', is sufficient. It is best not to say anything by way of self-justification or worse, self-praise. Let parents draw their own conclusions about the quality of care their baby has received. Do not expect to be appreciated too much at this point.

Depending on whether there has been any preparation for this moment or not and what state the mother is in physically, it is now almost always appropriate to let the parents hold their baby. Inasmuch as this is possible they need to be given time alone to grieve over their dead baby. Arrangements will be made for other family members to see and hold the baby according to parental wishes. Parents will often request the doctor to say a few words of explanation to relatives at this time.

Subsequent events

After this immediate grieving period the midwife or doctor should explain what comes next. The baby will be taken to the hospital mortuary. This often causes distress and parents quite frequently ask to see their baby again. Our experience is that if a post-mortem is thought necessary this is not the best time to ask. We normally (except in cultures where same-day burial is practised) arrange to see parents to provide the death certificate the following day and take that opportunity to make the request. Most units use a check list for perinatal deaths to ensure that all relevant professionals are informed, etc.

Other details

Living in such a heterogeneous society, it is not possible to cover every possible eventuality in this brief chapter. Nevertheless, consideration needs to be taken of a wide variation in nationality, language, religion, culture and even general life-style, all of which may profoundly affect the way neonatal deaths are approached. Neither doctors nor midwives are likely to have an encyclopaedic knowledge of these matters but, at the very least, it must be ensured that where there are language difficulties present a good translator is made available and that in the area of religion and culture, parents' wishes are actively sought and respected.

Chapter summary

The death of a baby is a very painful experience. As health professionals it is not possible to take the sting out of it but, by such simple, caring attention to detail as described in this chapter, it is possible to support parents through the crisis.

Chapter 16

Ethical and legal issues

Introduction

It is important to start resuscitation promptly and effectively when the need arises. However, it is equally important to recognize when these measures should be withheld or stopped. Consequently there are a number of ethical and legal issues faced by practitioners who are involved in newborn resuscitation. Sometimes difficult decisions have to be made and in the current NHS climate, with increasing risks of litigation, it is important for practitioners to ensure that they are able to justify their actions and provide a reasonable standard of care.

The purpose of this chapter is to discuss some of the ethical and legal issues in newborn resuscitation faced by medical and midwifery staff. It must be emphasized that only a brief insight into these issues can be provided in such a short chapter and further reading is essential if a comprehensive understanding is required or if policies and procedures need to be formulated.

Chapter objectives

At the end of this chapter the reader will be able to:

- discuss what is meant by a reasonable 'standard of care'
- discuss the criteria for deciding not to resuscitate
- discuss the criteria for not starting resuscitation and for stopping resuscitation
- discuss methods to manage the legal risks associated with newborn resuscitation.

Standard of care

A practitioner, e.g. a midwife or paediatrician, owes a 'duty of care' to a newborn baby in need of resuscitation, and is expected to provide a reasonable standard of care. Although at present there is little English precedent, it is quite possible, as has happened in the USA, that in the future patients and relatives may win claims for compensation for injury sustained during a resuscitation attempt if medical negligence can be proved. In the USA, birth-related complications constitute the largest single source of negligence against paediatricians (American Academy of Pediatrics, 1997).

The key issue applied by the courts when considering liability in medical negligence claims is an expectation that the patient should have received a reasonable standard of care. When determining whether this standard of care has been breached during any aspect of the resuscitation process, the level of experience and expertise that the practitioner has or is expected to have, together with the circumstances, will be taken into account.

'A claim of inexperience or lack of training will not be successful as defence in an allegation of negligence if a practitioner has been called upon only to work within the limits of his own expected competence' (Resuscitation Council (UK), 1998). On the other hand if 'an inexperienced practitioner is *obliged* to commence emergency treatment, but at the same time calls for specialist help, his lack of training will normally be a defence if his performance is sub-optimal' (Resuscitation Council (UK), 1998).

In the above circumstances the practitioner should bear in mind the likely availability of more skilled help and should exercise a cautious degree of intervention within the realms of their own skills and training.

It is also important to mention here, that where an expert practitioner takes control of a resuscitation procedure and delegates tasks to more junior members of staff within that team, that practitioner will remain accountable for any suboptimal treatment delivered by junior staff, if the same was outside their range of experience and training.

Although, in addition, where there is a reckless or negligent acceptance of a delegated task, there is liability on the practitioner who accepts that delegation where the result is harm to the patient.

In order to ascertain whether there has been a breach of duty, demonstrated by a failure in the standard of care delivered, it is first of all necessary to establish exactly what standard should have been followed and whether the defendant's actions differed to the patient's detriment, if at all, from what it was reasonable to expect (Dimond, 1994). The European Resuscitation Council (1998) and the Royal College of Paediatrics and Child Health (1997) have set a standard of care with the publication of their newborn resuscitation guidelines. It would be reasonable for the courts to expect medical and mid-wifery staff to ensure that they perform resuscitation to such a standard, within of course their capabilities and experience. 'It is important that practitioners should not take on responsibility beyond the level to which they have been trained' (Resuscitation Council (UK), 1998).

To determine the legal standard expected from practitioners, the courts use the so-called Bolam Test, which derives from a case decided in 1957. This 'Bolam standard' states that when you get a situation which involves the use of some special skill or competence, then the test as to where there has been negligence or not is ... the standard of the ordinary skilled man exercising and professing to have that special skill. A man need not possess the highest expert skill; it is well established that it is sufficient if he exercises the ordinary skill of an ordinary competent man exercising that particular art.

It was also stated in this case that, 'a doctor is not negligent if he is acting in accordance with a practice accepted as proper by a reasonable body of medical men skilled in that particular art, merely because there is a body of such opinion that takes a contrary view'. (The Bolam test of course applies to all health care practitioners and is not confined to medical staff.)

Therefore, the approach adopted by a practitioner during newborn resuscitation may not necessarily be regarded as negligent in all circumstances. However, deviating from nationally recognized guide-lines would require clear explanation and justification on the part of the practitioner involved should the patient suffer as a direct result.

When considering guidelines and protocols for resuscitation, the practitioner must always bear in mind the best interests of the patient. If applying a standard method of treatment supported by a protocol or guideline is clearly not relevant to the patient's needs and the same results in an adverse outcome for the patient, then the practitioner would be culpable under the Bolam principle. In the *Airdale Hospitals NHS Trust* v. *Bland* (1994) case, the court found that the medical staff who had followed the withdrawal of treatment guidelines published by the GMC were not negligent but only because the guidelines satisfied the Bolam test. The judges took pains to point out that had the guidelines not been in line with current accepted practice, the blind following of them would not have protected the Trust against a finding of negligence.

In the recent case of *Bolitho* v *City and Hackney Health Authority* (1998), the Court considered the sensibility of the application of the Bolam test for the first time since 1957. The judges held that it could not simply be the case that where there was support for a defendant doctor's actions through a responsible body of medical opinion, that doctor would not be negligent. The supporting opinion itself must be capable of logical analysis and common sense application.

For the Bolam test, this means that there is an additional criterion to a doctor not being negligent merely because there is a body of opinion with a contrary view. While this is still true, the converse is that a doctor may still be negligent *even* if there is a body of medical opinion which takes a supportive view unless that body of opinion can convince the court that it is reasonable in all the circumstances.

The important and new key is that, according to Dimond (1994), there are a number of lessons to be learnt from court cases in relation to an expected standard of care. Those that can be applied to newborn resuscitation are as follows:

- the practitioner must be familiar with the current standard of practice. This includes being aware of protocols, guidelines and procedures which have been drawn up both nationally and locally
- despite the availability of guidelines, there is still room for professional judgement and discretion. Clear and precise records must be kept which detail the particular circumstances and justification for departing from an agreed procedure
- the practitioner's knowledge and skills should be kept up-to-date because the standard of care will improve and the practitioner will be judged against the standard of the time, and not against the one applied several years earlier.

This standard of care is also expected from the Professional Bodies. In the Midwives' Code of Practice (UKCC, 1998b) it states that, 'you should be appropriately prepared and clinically up-to-date to ensure you are able effectively to carry out emergency procedures for the mother or baby such as resuscitation'. In addition, 'each practitioner retains the clinical accountability for her own practice'.

Failure to start resuscitation

Failing to start resuscitation when it is indicated would be considered negligent unless there is a:

- perceived risk – a practitioner may fail to start resuscitation if there is a perceived risk, e.g. having no ventilation device and facing the prospect of performing mouth-to-mouth resuscitation in an apnoeic newborn infant covered with amniotic fluid and blood, which would certainly be classed as an HIV risk. Although clearly the hospital is under a duty to ensure that all the necessary equipment is available.
- failure to recognize that the baby requires resuscitation – this is an unlikely defence however for most staff working with newborns. It is either a failure in training in which case the hospital could be seen to be negligent for failing to have skilled practitioners caring for vulnerable patients or, for medical and midwifery staff, who owe a duty of care to the baby, it would certainly be regarded as negligence.

When not to start resuscitation and when to stop resuscitation

Although present day expertise, knowledge, technology and pharmacology must undoubtedly improve the likelihood of successful resuscitation, there are times when it is futile and inhumane. If not indicated or unnecessarily prolonged, resuscitation can inflict an undignified death on the baby. Trying to determine the extent (if at all) and duration of resuscitation can sometimes be very difficult. A non-aggressive approach may on the one hand deny a baby a normal life, while on the other hand a prolonged and sustained resuscitation effort could result in a delayed death or the survival of a severely handicapped baby.

There are two specific ethical dilemmas which the practitioner may have to face:

- deciding not to start resuscitation (i.e. would be inappropriate)
- deciding when to stop when it is unsuccessful (i.e. it is inappropriate to continue).

Deciding not to start resuscitation

Sometimes difficult situations over whether to start resuscitation in the delivery room can arise unexpectedly following the birth of a very premature, ill or grossly deformed baby. The policy at most hospitals is to resuscitate all viable infants until the most appropriate correct course of action can be determined following a comprehensive assessment by a senior paediatrician and after discussion with the parents. Making a snap decision is not advisable, decisions should not be left to junior members of staff and the involvement of an experienced paediatrician is strongly recommended. It is also recommended that a senior paediatrician is present at the birth of an infant who is thought to be at the borderline of viability.

It is considered to be preferable to make a decision based on the gestational age rather than the birthweight (Royal College of Paediatrics and Child Health, 1997) because extreme growth-retarded infants have survived normally. It is important to discuss with the parents the possible need to restrict resuscitation measures at birth when severe perinatal problems are anticipated. All decisions should be documented in the mother's notes.

A difficult scenario arises where there are no fetal heart sounds prior to delivery, particularly when there is evidence of good outcomes following apparent stillbirths (Jain *et al.*, 1991). Some authorities recommend that resuscitation should be commenced if a fetal heart beat was detected up to 15 minutes prior to delivery (Milner, 1999). If in doubt err on the side of caution and begin resuscitation.

Deciding to stop resuscitation

Unfortunately, there is no firm evidence as to when resuscitation should be stopped, although the European Resuscitation Council (1998) does recommend that, 'resuscitation efforts should be discontinued if the baby does not have a cardiac output by 15 min or if the baby is failing to make any respiratory efforts despite naloxone therapy by 30 min'.

It is also worth noting that:

- if an infant has not established regular respirations following 30 minutes of effective resuscitation, the prognosis is very poor (Todres and Rogers, 1975)
- the need to administer adrenaline is associated with poor prognosis (Sims *et al.*, 1994).

Deciding not to start or deciding to stop resuscitation – who makes the decision?

Deciding when not to initiate resuscitation or indeed when to terminate a resuscitation attempt are two very difficult decisions for practitioners to make, particularly as the mother will be there in the room. They certainly should not be made by junior members of staff, but should be the responsibility of a senior member of staff, e.g. either a consultant or a specialist trainee paediatrician (Royal College of Paediatrics and Child Health, 1997).

It must be stressed that, 'all members of the clinical team should have an opportunity to voice their feelings' (Royal College of Paediatrics and Child Health, 1997a). So, although the senior paediatrician is ultimately responsible for making the decision to stop resuscitation, the team should always be consulted, as well as, of course, the parents. Clearly every situation should be assessed on an individual basis.

Risk management strategy

'Professionals can take a risk management approach to litigation which on the one hand ensures high standards of care and on the other high standards of evidence should litigation be threatened' (Henderson and Jones, 1997). Henderson and Jones (1997) suggest the following key components of a risk management strategy to minimize the risk of litigation:

- standards of care
- use of protocols
- monitoring practice
- identifying risk activities
- keeping records
- responding to complaints
- maintaining a safe environment.

Each will now be discussed in turn in the context of newborn resuscitation.

Standard of care

The law and the public will expect that the practitioner attains a recognized standard of care that would be expected from any competent healthcare professional. The practitioner will therefore need to keep up to date with current guidelines and strive to ensure that whenever possible practice is based on evidence. This will of course require not only knowledge but also, and just as importantly, competency at resuscitation skills. This is where, in particular, training and regular updates in resuscitation techniques are essential if this required level of competency is not only reached but maintained.

There should also be an audit system in place to ensure that these standards are being achieved and maintained. One possible and objective way of undertaking this is through scenario testing using a manikin, preferably in the clinical area, following recommended guidelines. It would certainly be more beneficial if the team approach to resuscitation is evaluated and it is therefore desirable to encourage participation of both the paediatrician and the midwife together which will help provide a realistic situation.

Protocols

These can help to reduce the risk of error and help to assure the desired standard of care and it is therefore important to ensure that protocols are established where they are needed, e.g. one recommending when a paediatrician should be present at the birth. Where appropriate, these protocols should be based on current research, guidelines and recommendations and they should be determined and agreed locally. It is important to ensure that all practitioners, who will be expected to follow them, are involved in their production. This will help to ensure that they are followed.

Monitoring practice

All resuscitation attempts should be audited. This can be done by either completing a standard audit form immediately following the event (preferable) or retrospectively by reviewing the infant's notes. The main purpose of the audit is to identify any problems, e.g. with equipment or with the resuscitation procedure and to rectify them accordingly. In addition, potential problems can also be highlighted.

Identifying risk activities

In particular, interpretation of meconium staining, decisions on when to request medical support and resuscitation are areas of clinical practice which are prone to or favour successful litigation (Henderson and Jones, 1997). Again it is important to ensure that regular training is undertaken and appropriate protocols not only in place but also reviewed.

Keeping records

The keeping of clear comprehensive records is part of the duty of care owed to the client (Dimond, 1994). In addition they are invaluable in the providing of evidence in cases of litigation. It is therefore imperative to ensure that high standards of record keeping are maintained. It is worth noting that there are national guidelines on record keeping, e.g. the UKCC's 'Standards for Records and Record Keeping' (1993).

Responding to complaint

It is clearly preferable to deal with complaints at an early stage so as to prevent them from turning into a formal complaint. In addition, good communication and explanations, and involving the parents in the decision making, may also reduce the incidence of complaints in the first place.

Maintaining a safe environment

The requirements of the Health and Safety at Work Act (1974) should of course be followed. Care should particularly be taken with sharps and body fluids. Regular checks should be carried out on the resuscitation equipment following the manufacturers' recommendations and any faults or defects reported and rectified.

Conclusion

If resuscitation is required it is essential to start promptly and effectively. However, it is just as important to recognize when these measures should be withheld or stopped. The practitioner must be aware of these ethical and legal dilemmas and ensure that a reasonable standard of care is provided in newborn resuscitations.

Chapter 17

Training issues

Introduction

Newborn resuscitation requires skills that are essentially practical and practitioners need hands-on practical training to acquire and maintain them. Formal training is rarely possible in the clinical area. Fortunately, however, it is now possible, with modern training manikins and models, to provide realistic training using simulations and scenarios.

The aim of this chapter is to identify the training requirements for different staff groups based on national guidelines and discuss how this training can be best provided and evaluated.

Chapter objectives

At the end of the chapter the reader will be able to:

- discuss why resuscitation training is important
- discuss the proposals of the Joint Standing Committee Report 'The Training Needs of Professionals Responsible for Resuscitation of Babies at Birth'
- discuss various methods of resuscitation training
- discuss the evaluation of resuscitation training.

Resuscitation training – why it is important

Poor resuscitation skills

It is well documented that practitioners' skills in paediatric and adult resuscitation are often very poor (Lowenstein *et al.*, 1981; Wynne *et al.*, 1987; Buss *et al.*, 1993). Poor skills in newborn resuscitation are also prevalent. The 1998 Confidential Enquiry into Stillbirths and Deaths in Infancy Report stated that:

- a junior paediatrician was unable to intubate a baby on four occasions. 'This removed any chance the baby might have had'
- problems with resuscitation were identified in 60% of the reported cases of asphyxia.

Perceived and actual competence at resuscitation

- There is considerable disparity between perceived competence and the actual ability to undertake effective resuscitation (Smith and Hatchett, 1992).
- Experience of senior practitioners attending cardiac arrests is that confidence levels are often high but this is often not matched by high skill levels (Wynne *et al.*, 1987).
- The fact that practitioners are unable accurately to assess their own competence reinforces the argument that resuscitation training and regular updates should be compulsory for all practitioners regardless of their seniority and experience.

Retention of skills

- Retention of resuscitation skills is very poor (McKenna and Glendon, 1985; Moser and Coleman, 1992).
- A significant deterioration in competence has been shown after only 10 weeks (Broomfield, 1996).

Resuscitation training – national recommendations and guidelines

There is a definite need for resuscitation training and re-training. This has been recognized by the Royal Colleges in their recent publications (British Paediatric Association, 1993; Royal College of Paediatrics and Child Health, 1997). In addition, the *Fifth Annual Report of the Confidential Enquiry into Stillbirths and Deaths in Infancy (1998)* has emphasized the importance of ensuring that practitioners present at birth are proficient in newborn resuscitation.

In 1997 the Joint Standing Committee RCPCH/RCOG published their document 'The Training Needs of Professionals Responsible for Resuscitation of Babies at Birth' (Royal College of Paediatrics and Child Health, 1997). The following recommendations were made.

Joint Standing Committee RCPCH/RCOG's 'The Training Needs of Professionals Responsible for Resuscitation of Babies at Birth' (1997)

This document has been approved by both the councils of the Royal College of Obstetricians and Gynaecologists and the Royal College of Paediatrics and Child Health. In addition it has been endorsed by:

- British Association of Perinatal Medicine
- Neonatal Nurses Association
- Royal College of Anaesthetists
- Royal College of Midwives.

The document describes the training and assessment needs of all practitioners who may be involved with newborn resuscitation, including nurses, midwives, neonatal nurses, paediatricians, anaesthetists, obstetricians and general practitioners.

Level of training required

The document identifies four broad categories of staff:

- novices
- trainees
- staff with responsibility for suction
- experienced staff.

It describes the essential training needs for each one. These recommendations should be considered as guidance from which individual training needs can be determined and training then provided based on local requirements. Each staff group will now be discussed in turn in respect of the recommendations.

Novices

(Students and those transferring to work in the delivery suite, but not expected to be responsible for resuscitation, e.g. student nurses, medical students.)

Background reading is essential and should be readily available. In addition novices should:

- attend lectures covering the physiology and biochemistry of the adaptation to extrauterine life
- attend neonatal resuscitation training sessions which should be practically oriented using manikins and simulations
- receive training in effective airway management, bag/valve/mask ventilation and chest compressions
- observe experienced practitioners carrying out resuscitation procedures
- be familiar with the unit guidelines and procedures for newborn resuscitation.

Trainees
(Qualified staff in junior positions who are working in departments where there will always be experienced staff immediately available.)

As well as the training needs highlighted above for novices, trainees should:

- assist with resuscitation procedures
- have specific training needs for their post and responsibilities identified.

Staff with responsibility for resuscitation
(All midwives, those responsible for home deliveries including general practitioners, senior house officers and specialist registrars in obstetrics, paediatrics and anaesthetics, neonatal nurses and practitioners.)

All staff with responsibility for resuscitation should have:

- revision and appraisal of all skills previously acquired
- training with supervised practice
- regular audit of skills and training and dissemination of information.

Experienced staff
(Specialist registrars in paediatrics and neonatology, staff grade and consultant paediatricians, and other practitioners who have positions of responsibility for newborn resuscitation including obstetricians, anaesthetists, midwives, neonatal nurses and practitioners.)

All experienced staff should:

- have skills regularly revised
- be trained in endotracteal intubation with both practice and supervision
- be trained in umbilical venous catheterization
- be trained in the appropriate use of drugs
- supervise novices, trainees and staff with responsibilities for resuscitation
- play an active role in teaching
- assume responsibility for the organization and audit of skills and training.

Resuscitation training – methods

Although considerable research has been undertaken evaluating the principles of teaching adult basic and advanced resuscitation skills, there is very little in the literature evaluating the teaching of newborn resuscitation. However, the same principles of teaching adult resuscitation could be applied to the teaching of newborn resuscitation. The fundamentals of resuscitation training and retention of skills will now be discussed.

Factors affecting skill attainment and skill retention

- Both course content and time devoted to practice on manikins will influence skill attainment and subsequent retention of skills (Wynne, 1995).
- Constructive feedback during training is important and should not only identify the student's strong points, which will clearly increase their confidence and motivation, but also should identify any weaknesses or deficiencies which need to be addressed and require more practice.

Lectures

Lectures can:

- be used to revise core material and highlight key points
- complement practical stations, but should not replace practical teaching on manikins and models

- provide an opportunity for group discussion
- help maintain interest, the lecturer should remember the following key points: conciseness, simplicity, eye contact, variations in speed and volume and the use of personal experience and questions (Advanced Life Support Group, 1999).

Skill stations

As resuscitation involves essentially practical skills, it is therefore important to ensure that any training session allocates plenty of time for these practical skills to be taught and practised. Skill stations should:

- provide an opportunity to learn a skill and debate relevant issues
- be put into the context of the resuscitation procedure
- be undertaken in small groups
- take into account, and build on, prior experience and knowledge. Shared aspects of teaching, learning and prior experience will promote both positive regard and mutual respect
- provide positive feedback. Encouragement and guidance are particularly important when teaching practical skills.

The Advanced Life Support Group (1999) suggest a four stage approach to the teaching of practical skills.

Four stage approach to teaching a practical skill

- Instructor demonstrates the skill silently (silent run through). The skill is carried out at normal speed without explanation and commentary, except what would normally be said in the clinical situation. This allows the student to carefully observe the procedure without distraction.
- Instructor demonstrates the skill again, but this time with a commentary. The skill is demonstrated again, but this time with explanation and will be broken down into small steps. It will generally not be at normal speed.
- Student provides the commentary while the instructor demonstrates the skill. This stage is used because a skill is more likely to be learned if the student can describe it in detail (The Advanced Life Support Group (1999). If the student is hesitant, the instructor can prompt by leading with the actions. On the other hand, confident candidates can describe the different stages of the

skill before they are demonstrated. Any errors must be corrected immediately.

- Student demonstrates the skill together with a commentary. Each student talks through and demonstrates the skill. The instructor now has an opportunity to observe each student and ensure that they have understood and also are competent at the skill.

Scenarios

The purpose of resuscitation training is to teach the trainees to resuscitate newborn babies and therefore any teaching method that can help to simulate the real situation will facilitate both teaching and assessment. The scenario is a simulated resuscitation attempt that involves all the practitioners who would be involved with newborn resuscitation in integrating and practising their resuscitation skills in their individual roles. It can form a major part of any training session and it logically follows on from the teaching and practice of individual skills, e.g. face mask resuscitation and chest compressions. It is a way of putting it all together in a systematic and meaningful way.

There are numerous advantages to this form of training:

- ideal for training in the clinical area
- can help effectively to evaluate both an individual and a group performance (Kaye and Mancini, 1986)
- allows practitioners the opportunity to practise their skills and to learn to work together in a coordinated fashion
- can help to bridge the theory/practice gap
- can increase efficiency and credibility, improve communication and decision making and reduce anxiety (Wynne, 1995).

Key learning objectives

Detailed below is a suggested list of key learning objectives which may help in the provision of training in newborn resuscitation:

- demonstrate correct procedure for checking emergency equipment
- discuss the importance of minimizing heat loss and preventing cold stress
- discuss the initial evaluation of a newborn infant
- state the correct procedure for summoning senior help
- demonstrate two safe methods of tactile stimulation

- demonstrate the correct procedure for opening and maintaining a clear airway
- specify the indications for face mask resuscitation
- demonstrate the correct procedure for face mask resuscitation
- specify the indications for the need to start chest compressions
- demonstrate two safe methods of chest compressions
- specify the indications for intubation
- list the equipment required for intubation
- demonstrate a correct and safe procedure for intubation
- list four complications of intubation
- describe the two common routes for drug administration
- specify the indications for administering adrenaline
- discuss when resuscitation should be abandoned
- discuss the possible indications for withholding resuscitation measures
- discuss the process of constant re-assessment during a resuscitation attempt
- describe how the parents can receive support during a resuscitation attempt.

Provision of resuscitation training

Most hospitals provide in-house training in newborn resuscitation which is tailored to meet local needs and follows national guidelines and recommendations. It is preferable if this training is practically oriented using manikins and models as appropriate.

Evaluation of resuscitation training/courses

All courses and training sessions should be continually evaluated to determine whether learning objectives have been met and whether the teaching format is appropriate.

There is, without doubt, value in auditing resuscitation skills and decision making in the clinical area using scenarios (simulated resuscitations). Bishop-Kurylo and Masiello (1995) developed a mock code programme and evaluation tool to assess and enhance the competency of both nursing and medical staff who respond to paediatric arrests. They evaluated all the critical skills required for paediatric resuscitation and the tool not only identifies educational requirements but also problems with the resuscitation equipment and procedures.

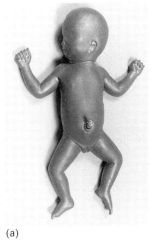

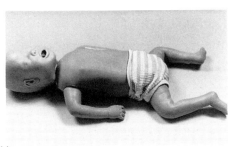

(b)

(a)

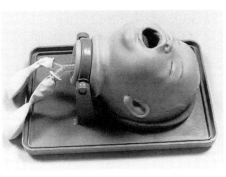

Fig. 17.1   (a), (b) and (c)
Training manikins and
models   (c)

Recognized courses

Resuscitation Council (UK) NALS Course

The Resuscitation Council (UK) approved Neonatal Advanced Life
Support Course (NALS) is run by a few centres. It is a two-day
practically oriented course and covers important aspects of neonatal
resuscitation. For further information contact the Resuscitation
Council (UK) on 0207 388 4678.

American Academy of Pediatrics Neonatal Resuscitation Program

This one-day course, which is overseen by the American Academy of
Pediatrics, is offered by only a few centres in the UK. For further
information contact Phil Jevon at the Manor Hospital, Walsall,
Tel. 01922 656367.

Training manikins/models (Fig. 17.1)

There are a number of infant airway management manikins available. Most are anatomically correct in size and detail and benefit from having realistic landmarks including nostrils, tongue, oro- and nasopharynx, larynx, epiglottis, vocal cords, trachea, oesophagus, inflatable lungs and stomach.

Airway management skills that can be demonstrated and practised include the sizing and insertion of Guedal airways, suction and intubation. However, it is not possible on some of the manikins realistically to perform face mask ventilation as the maintenance of an open airway is not always necessary to achieve chest rise. An infant manikin is a better alternative.

Chapter summary

The importance of resuscitation training has been discussed. The national recommendations for training have been outlined and the various methods of resuscitation training including training equipment has been described. Retention of skills is poor and regular re-training and experience are required to ensure that competence is maintained at a satisfactory level.

References

Adamsons K Jr *et al.* (1965) The influence of thermal factors upon oxygen consumption of the newborn human infant. *Journal of Pediatrics*, **66**, 495–508.

Advanced Life Support Group (1999) *Pocket Guide to Teaching for Medical Instructors.* BMJ, London.

American Academy of Pediatrics (1996) *Neonatal Resuscitation.* American Academy of Pediatrics, USA.

American Heart Association and American Academy of Pediatrics (1997) *Pediatric Advanced Life Support.* American Heart Association, USA.

Apgar V (1953) The proposal for a new method of evaluation of the newborn infant. *Anaesthetic Analgesia*, **32**, 260–267.

Arieff AI, Leach W, Park R *et al.* (1982) Systemic effects of $NaHCO_3$ in experimental lactic acidosis in dogs. *American Journal of Physiology*, **242**, F586–F591.

Berkowitz ID, Chantarojanasira T, Koehler RC *et al.* (1989) Blood flow during cardiopulmonary resuscitation with simultaneous compression and ventilation in pigs. *Pediatric Research*, **26**, 558–564.

Booth P (1996) *The Handbook of Neonatal Transport: A Practical Approach for Scotland.* Neonatal Unit, Aberdeen Maternity Hospital.

Bishop-Kurylo D, Masiello M (1995) Pediatric resuscitation: development of a mock code program and evaluation tool. *Pediatric Nursing*, **21**, 333–336.

Bolam v Friern Hospital Management Committee (1957) in Dimond B (1994) *The Legal Aspects of Midwifery.* Books for Midwifery Press, Cheshire.

Broomfield R (1996) A quasi-experimental research to investigate the retention of basic cardiopulmonary resuscitation skills and knowledge by qualified nurses following a course in professional development. *Journal of Advanced Nursing*, **23**, 1016–1023.

British Paediatric Association (1993) *The Report of a BPA Working Party Group.* British Paediatric Association, London.

Bryan E (1992) *Twins and Higher Multiple Births.* Edward Arnold, London.

Buss PW, McCabe M, Evans RJ *et al.* (1993) A survey of basic resuscitation knowledge among resident paediatricians. *Archives of Disease in Childhood*, **68**, 75–78.

Chernow B, ed. (1988) *The Pharmacological Approach to the Critically Ill Patient*, 2nd edn. Baltimore, MD: Williams & Wilkins: 486–487.

Codero L, How EH (1971) Neonatal bradycardia following nasopharyngeal suction. *Journal of Pediatrics*, **78**, 441.

Confidential Enquiry into Stillbirths and Deaths in Infancy (1998) *Fifth Annual Report*. Maternal and Child Health Research Consortium, London.

David R (1988) Closed chest cardiac massage in the newborn infant. *Paediatrics*, **81**, 552–554.

Davies J, Hey E, Reid W *et al.* (1996) Prospective regional study of planned home birth. *British Medical Journal*, **313**, 1302–1305.

Dawes GS (1968) *Fetal and Neonatal Physiology*. Year Book Medical Publishers Inc, Chicago, Chapter 12.

Department of Health (1993) *Changing Childbirth*. HMSO, London.

Dimond B (1994) *The Legal Aspects of Midwifery*. Books for Midwifery Press, Cheshire.

Duffy TE, Kohle SJ, Vannucci RC (1975) Carbohydrate and energy metabolism in perinatal rat brain: relation to survival in anoxia. *Journal of Neurochemistry*, **24**, 271–276.

Ellemunter H, Simma B, Trawoger R *et al.* (1999) Intraosseous lines in preterm and full term neonates. *Archives of Disease in Childhood, Fetal Neonatal Edition*, **80**, F74–F75.

European Resuscitation Council (1998) *The 1998 European Resuscitation Council Guidelines for Resuscitation of Babies at Birth* in *European Resuscitation Council Guidelines for Resuscitation*, Elsevier, Oxford.

Finberg L (1977) The relationship of intravenous infusion and intracranial hemorrhage: a commentary. *Journal of Pediatrics*, **91**, 777.

Gandy GM, Adamson K, Cunningham N *et al.* (1964) Thermal environment and acid–base homeostasis in human infants during the first few hours of life. *Journal of Clinical Investigation*, **43**, 751–758.

Gazmuri RJ, von Planta M, Weil MH *et al.* (1990) Cardiac effects of carbon dioxide–consuming and carbon dioxide-generating buffers during cardiopulmonary resuscitation. *Journal of the American College of Cardiology*, **15**, 482–490.

Ginsberg HD, Goldsmith JP (1998) Controversies in neonatal resuscitation. *Clinics in Perinatology*, 25, no 1 March.

Handal KA, Schauben JL, Salamone FR *et al.* (1983) Naloxone. *Annals of Emergency Medicine*, **12**, 438–445.

Health and Safety at Work Act (1974) HMSO, London.

Henderson C, Jones K (1997) *Essential Midwifery*. Mosby, London.

Hey EN (1969) The relation between environmental temperature and oxygen consumption in the newborn baby. *Journal of Physiology*, **200**, 589–603.

Howell J (1987) Sodium bicarbonate in the perinatal setting revisited. *Clinical Perinatology*, **14**, 807–816.

Jain L, Ferre C, Vidyasagar D *et al.* (1991) Cardiopulmonary resuscitation of apparently stillborn infants: survival and long-term outcome. *Journal of Pediatrics*, **118**, 778.

Kaye W, Mancini ME (1986) Use of the Mega Code to evaluate team leader performance during advanced cardiac life support. *Critical Care Medicine*, **14**, 99–104.

Klaus MH, Kennel JH (1976) *Maternal Infant Bonding*. Mosby, St Louis.

Laerdal (1997) *Laerdal Silicone Resuscitators, Directions for Use*. Laerdal, Orpington, Kent.

Lancet (1989) Breath of life. **1**, 305–306.

Langham Jr. MR, Kays DW, Ledbetter DJ *et al.* (1996) Congenital diaphragmatic hernia: epidemiology and outcome. *Clinical Perinatology,* **23**, 671–688.

Leslie AJ, Stephenson TJ (1998) Transporting sick newborn babies. *Current Paediatrics,* **8**, 98–102.

Lindemann R (1984) Resuscitation of the newborn. Endotracheal administration of epinephrine. *Acta Paediatrica Scandinavica,* **73**, 210–212.

Lowenstein SR, Libby L, Mountain R *et al.* (1981) Cardiopulmonary resuscitation of medical and surgical house officers. *Lancet,* **2**, 679–681.

McKenna SP, Glendon AI (1985) Occupational first aid training. Decay in CPR skills. *Journal of Occupational Psychology,* **58**, 109–117.

Mann TP (1968) Observations on temperatures of mothers and babies in the perinatal period. *Journal of Obstetrics and Gynaecology of the British Commonwealth,* **75**, 316–321.

Michael JR, Guerci AD, Koehler RC *et al.* (1984) Mechanisms by which epinephrine augments cerebral and myocardial perfusion during cardiopulmonary resuscitation in dogs. *Circulation,* **69**, 822–835.

Milner AD (1991) Resuscitation of the newborn. *Archives of Diseases in Childhood,* **66**, 66–69.

Milner AD (1998) Resuscitation at birth. *European Journal of Pediatrics,* **157**, 524–527.

Milner AD, (1999) Resuscitation at birth. In *ABC of Resuscitation* (MC Colquhoun, AJ Handley, TR Evans eds). BMJ Books, London.

Moser DK, Coleman S (1992) Recommendations for improving cardiopulmonary resuscitation skills retention. *Heart and Lung,* **21**, 372–380.

Murray Parkes C (1986) *Bereavement. Studies of Grief in Adult Life,* 2nd edn. Routledge, London.

Northern Neonatal Network (1996) *Principles of Neonatal Resuscitation,* 4th edn. Royal Victoria Infirmary, Newcastle-upon-Tyne.

North West Thames Health Authority *North West Thames Annual Maternity Figures (1992 and 1993)* London.

Office for National Statistics (1994) *Birth Statistics.* HMSO, London.

Ostrea EM Jr, Odell GB (1972) The influence of bicarbonate administration on blood pH in a 'closed' system: clinical implications. *Journal of Pediatrics,* **80**, 671.

Palme C, Nystrom B, Tunell R (1985) An evaluation of the efficiency of face masks in the resuscitation of newborn infants. *Lancet,* **1**, 207–210.

Papile LA, Burstein J, Burstein R *et al.* (1978) Relationship of intravenous sodium bicarbonate infusion and cerebral intraventricular hemorrhage. *Journal of Pediatrics,* **93**, 834.

Pasternak JF,Groothius DR, Fischer JM *et al.* (1983) Regional cerebral blood flow in the beagle puppy model of neonatal intraventricular hemorrhage: studies during systemic hypertension. *Neurology,* **33**, 559.

Perlman JM, Reiser R (1995) Cardiopulmonary resuscitation in the delivery room. *Archives of Pediatric and Adolescent Medicine,* **149**, 20.

Phillips G, Zideman DA (1986) Relation of infant heart to sternum: its significance in cardiopulmonary resuscitation. *Lancet,* **1**, 1024–1025.

Ramji S, Ahuja S, Thiupuram S *et al.* (1993) Resuscitation of asphyxic newborn infants with room air or 100% oxygen. *Pediatric Research,* **34**,

809–812.

Resuscitation Council (UK) (1998) *Advanced Life Support Course Provider Manual*. Resuscitation Council (UK), London.

Roberton NRC (1996) *A Manual of Normal Neonatal Care*, 2nd edn. Edward Arnold, London.

Royal College of Paediatrics and Child Health (1997) *Resuscitation of Babies at Birth*. BMJ Publishing Group, London.

Rutter N, Hull D (1979) Water loss from the skin of term and preterm babies. *Archives of Diseases in Childhood*, **54**, 858–868.

Sims DG, Heal CA, Bartle SM (1994) The use of adrenaline and atropine in neonatal resuscitation. *Archives of Diseases in Childhood*, **70**, F3–F10.

Smith S, Hatchett R (1992) Perceived competence in cardiopulmonary resuscitation, knowledge and skills, amongst 50 qualified nurses. *Intensive and Critical Care Nursing*, **8**, 76–81.

Speidel B, Fleming P, Henderson J (1998) *A Neonatal Vade-Mecum*, 3rd edn. Edward Arnold, London.

Stephenson JM, Du JN, Oliver TK (1970) The effect of cooling on blood gas tensions in newborn infants. *Journal of Pediatrics*, **76**, 848–852.

Stewart A and Dent A (1994) *At a Loss. Bereavement Care When a Baby Dies*.

Todres ID, Rogers MC (1975) Methods of external cardiac massage in the newborn infant. *Pediatrics*, **86**, 781–782.

UKCC (1993) *Standards for Records and Record Keeping*. UKCC, London.

UKCC (1998a) *Guidelines for records and record keeping*. UKCC, London.

UKCC (1998b) *Midwife's Rules and Code of Practice*. UKCC, London.

Vyas H, Milner AD, Hopkin IE *et al.* (1981) Physiologic responses to prolonged slow rise inflation in the resuscitation of the asphyxiated newborn infant. *Journal of Pediatrics*, **99**, 635–639.

Whyte SD, Sinha AJ, Wyllie JP (1998) Inability to adhere to current European Neonatal Resuscitation guidelines. *Resuscitation*, **37**, S62.

Whyte SD, Sinha AJ, Wyllie JP (1999) Neonatal resuscitation – a practical assessment. *Resuscitation*, **40**, 21–25.

Winkler CL, Hauth JC, Gilstrap LC III *et al.* (1991) Neonatal complications at term as related to the degree of umbilical arterial acidemia. *American Journal of Obstetrics and Gynecology*, **164**, 637.

Wiswell TE, Tuggle JM, Turner BS (1990) Meconium aspiration syndrome: have we made a difference? *Pediatrics*, **85**, 715–721.

Wynne G, Marteau TM, Johnston M *et al.* (1987) Inability of trained nurses to perform basic life support. *British Medical Journal*, **294**, 1198–1199.

Wynne G (1995) Training and retention of skills. In *ABC of Resuscitation* (MC Colquhoun, AJ Handley, TR Evans eds). BMJ Books, London.

Yeo H (1998) *Nursing the Neonate*. Blackwell Science, London.

Index